#1

www.CrosswordWeaver.com

ACROSS

2 canal, duct
3 occuring in an abnormal position
7 binary compound of oxygen with an element or chemical group
9 of, relating to, affecting or involving an ovary
11 inflammatory condition of the skin

DOWN

1 one of three divisions of the psyche in psychoanalytic theory
2 resembling mucous
4 a salt or ester of tartaric acid
5 twitching
6 carrying or propagating infection
8 shaped like an egg
10 an anatomical vessel :duct

#2

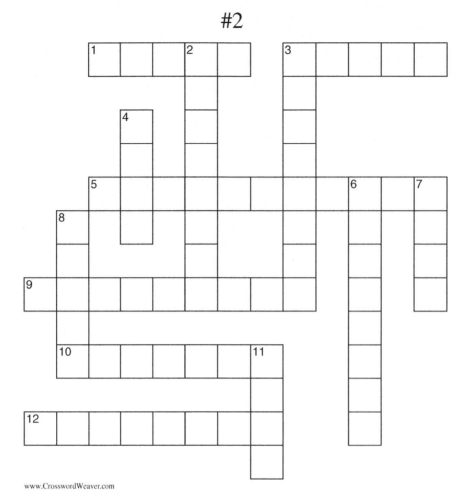

www.CrosswordWeaver.com

ACROSS

1 to make an effort to vomit
3 position in a chromosome of a particular gene or allele
5 marked interest in excrement
9 hemiplegia plus paralysis of a limb on the opposite side
10 an abnormal particle (as an air bubble) circulating in the blood
12 discharge from the external ear

DOWN

2 to deprive of testes
3 malignant tumor of lymphoid tissue
4 smallest part of an element
6 a filament (as a thread) used in surgery for tying blood vessels
7 fever marked by paroxysms of chills and sweating that recurs at regular intervals
8 to have or cause strong and repeated emptying of the bowels
11 to remove the ovaries and uterus of an animal

#3

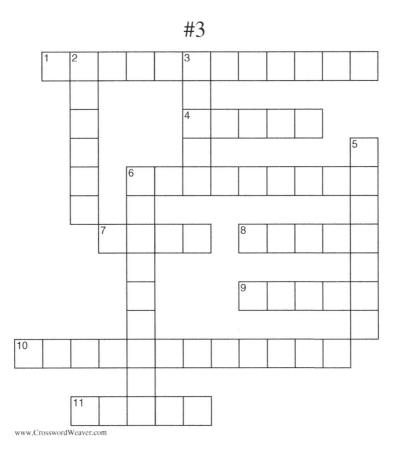

www.CrosswordWeaver.com

ACROSS

1 condition characterized by decrease in bone mass with decreased density and enlargement of bone spaces producing porosity and fragility
4 any of several diseases caused by skin lesions
6 a state of feeling unwell or unhappy
7 a skin sore caused by chronic irritation
8 a poisonous protein in the castor bean
9 relating to, involving, affecting, or located in the region of the kidneys
10 surgical removal of the pineal gland
11 a fold of mucous membrane partly or wholly closing the orifice of the vagina

DOWN

2 of, relating to, or lying near the sacrum
3 a hair or a structure resembling a hair
5 a small tube for insertion into a body cavity, duct, or vessel
6 body partition of muscle and connective tissue separating chest and abdominal cavities

#4

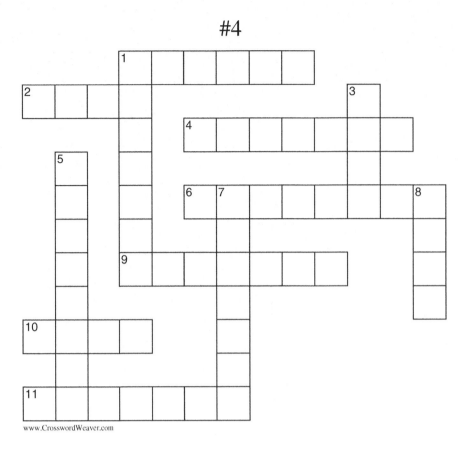

www.CrosswordWeaver.com

ACROSS

1 outer or superficial part of an organ or body structure

2 the bone on the little-finger side of the forearm that forms with the humerus the elbow joint

4 difficult or labored respiration

6 occuring over a wide geographic area and affecting an exceptionally high proportion of the population

9 small collapsible tube fitted with a hypodermic needle for injecting a single dose of a medicinal agent

10 an individual into which a tissue or part is transplanted from another

11 loss of thirst

DOWN

1 either of the angles formed by the meeting of the upper and lower eyelids

3 a microorganism causing disease

5 any of various synthetic or naturally occuring analogs of vitamin A

7 the absense or impairment of the sense of taste

8 coagulated mass produced by clotting of blood

#5

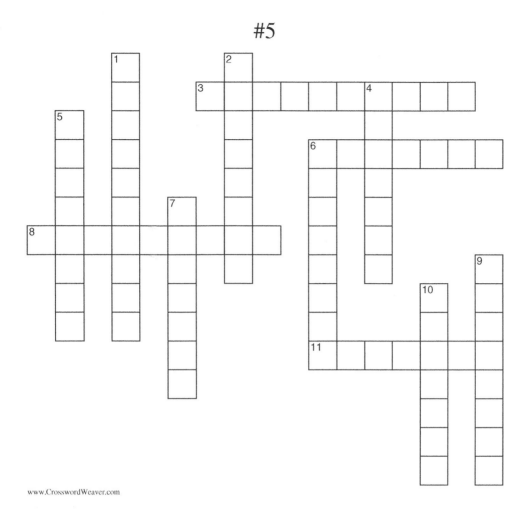

www.CrosswordWeaver.com

ACROSS

3 stoppage or sluggishness of blood flow

6 of, or relating to, or affected with jaundice

8 inflammation of the mucous membrane of the stomach

11 a tumor that arises from the tissue elements of the thymus

DOWN

1 the surgical removal of part of the iris of the eye

2 death of living tissue

4 examination of the body after death

5 of or relating to the mouth and nose

6 a homograft between genetically identical individuals

7 a brittle greyish white chiefly trivalent metallic element

9 the beginning of the menstrual function

10 of or relating to the tongue

#6

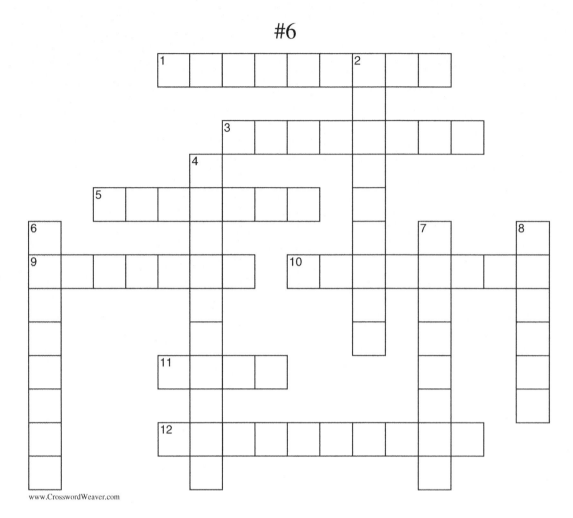

www.CrosswordWeaver.com

ACROSS

1 to put into a state of narcosis
3 inflammation of the uterus
5 of, relating to, or composed of bone
9 deficiency of oxygen reaching the tissues of the body
10 disorder of muscle tissue or muscles
11 devoid of sensation
12 compulsive eating of ice:symptom of lack of iron

DOWN

2 the study of the iris of the eye
4 occurring about or surrounding nervous tissue or a nerve
6 an enzyme that facilitates the clotting of blood
7 of, relating to, or affected by rickets
8 cell formed by union of two gametes

#7

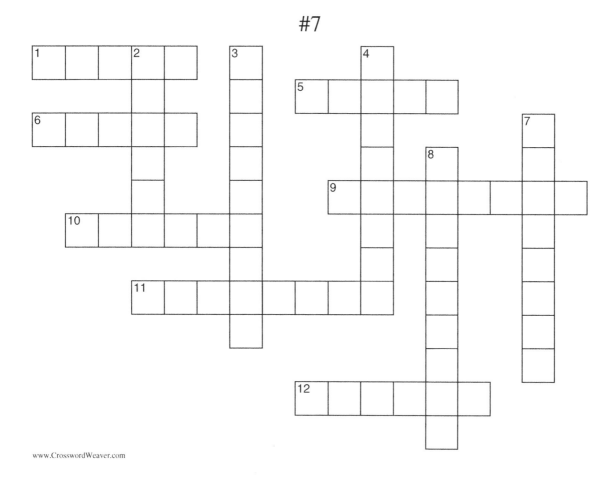

ACROSS

1 belch
5 anatomical pit or depression
6 abnormal excess accumulation of serous fluid in connective tissue or in a serous cavity
9 a malignant tumor of the renal cortex
10 situated opposite to or away from the mouth
11 urination at night : esp. when excessive
12 a discharge from the uterus and vagina following delivery

DOWN

2 blackhead
3 a urinary calculus
4 an abnormally watery state of the blood
7 a mass of clotted blood that forms in a tissue, organ, or body space as a result of a broken blood vessel
8 inflammation of the lip

#8

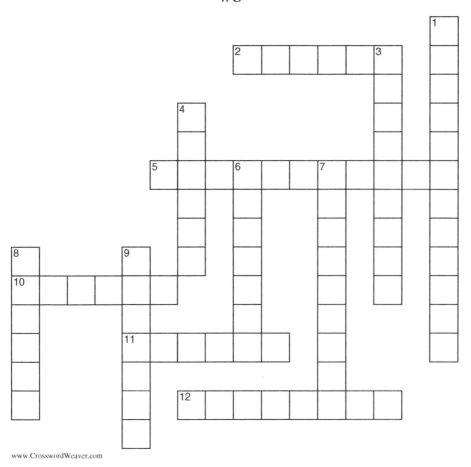

www.CrosswordWeaver.com

ACROSS

2 being in a normal or abnormal state of distension:swollen

5 obsession with and erotic interest in or stimulation by corpses

10 bedbug

11 first digit of the forelimb

12 to dry up or cause to dry up

DOWN

1 condition of containing more than the normal amount of acid

3 soft like mush

4 a small hammer with a rubber head used in medicinal percussion

6 the tearing apart of a tissue

7 abnormally low pressure of the intraocular fluid

8 not manifest or detectable by clinical methods alone

9 condition of carbon dioxide deficiency in blood and tissues

#9

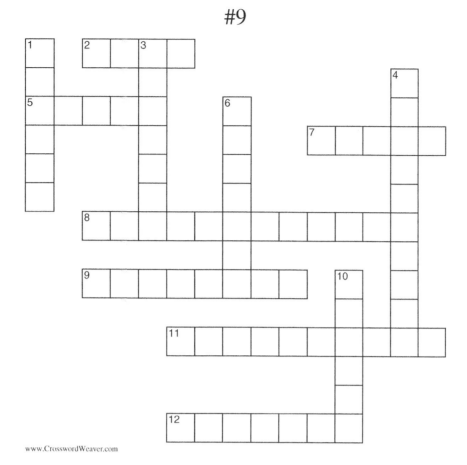

www.CrosswordWeaver.com

ACROSS

2 abnormal sound heard accompanying the normal respiratory sounds on auscultation of the chest
5 a red blood cell that has lost its hemoglobin
7 device worn to reduce a hernia by pressure
8 hemorrhage into the spinal cord
9 to waste away physically
11 having a common placenta---used of multiple fetuses
12 the inner or deep part of an organ or structure

DOWN

1 a cell formed by the union of two gametes
3 soft silver-white element that is the lightest metal known
4 impairment of the ability to write caused by brain damage
6 a nodular lesion of leprosy
10 acute inflammatory contagious disease involving the upper respiratory tract

#10

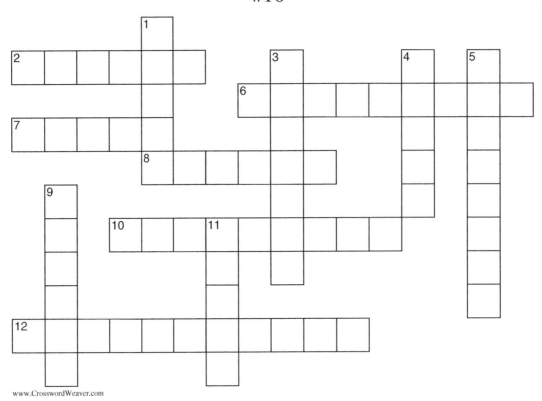

www.CrosswordWeaver.com

ACROSS

2 an agent that induces vomiting
6 dread of or aversion to novelty
7 a disturbed state of consciousness in which the one affected seems to perform acts in full awareness but upon recovery cannot recollect them
8 cancellous bony tissue between the external and internal layers of the skull
10 inflammation of the glans penis
12 profuse perspiration artificially induced

DOWN

1 a two footed animal
3 abnormal dryness of a body part or tissue (as the skin)
4 an official or standard collection of drug formulas and descriptions
5 a disorder of vision in which two images of a single object are seen
9 shaped approximately like a cube
11 to stop in the early stages

#11

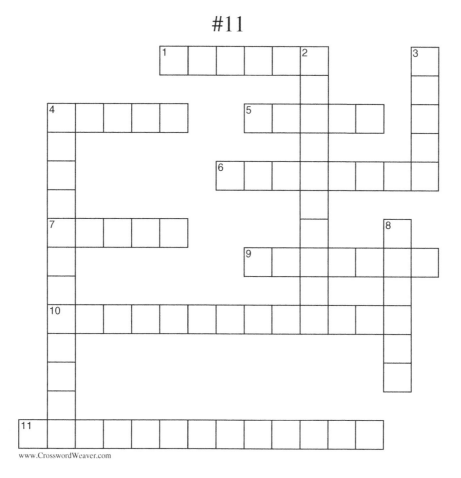

www.CrosswordWeaver.com

ACROSS

1 a scale or flake (as of skin)
4 a pinching spasmodic intestinal pain
5 to ooze or cause to ooze out
6 eyelid
7 a painful spasmodic condition of muscles (as of the neck or back)
9 a muscle that raises or keeps a part erect
10 backward flow of blood through a defective heart valve
11 plastic surgery to repair laryngeal defects

DOWN

2 having effects or capacities
3 transient cessation of respiration
4 spontaneous flow of milk from the nipple
8 a depressant drug

#12

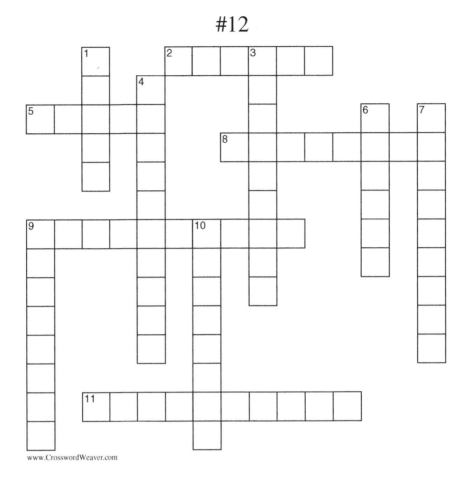

www.CrosswordWeaver.com

ACROSS

2 the upper surface of an appendage or part
5 of or relating to the cheek, the side of the head, or the zygomatic bone
8 having or growing in a form like that of a cluster of grapes
9 moving or tending to move the eyeball
11 heartburn

DOWN

1 the inward curved rim of the external ear
3 secreting sebum
4 surgical opening of the skull
6 an inanimate object (as a dish or clothing) that may be contaminated with infectious organisms and serve in their transmission
7 a state or period during which the symptoms of a disease are abated
9 a discharge from the external ear
10 a support or brace for weak or ineffective joints or muscles

#13

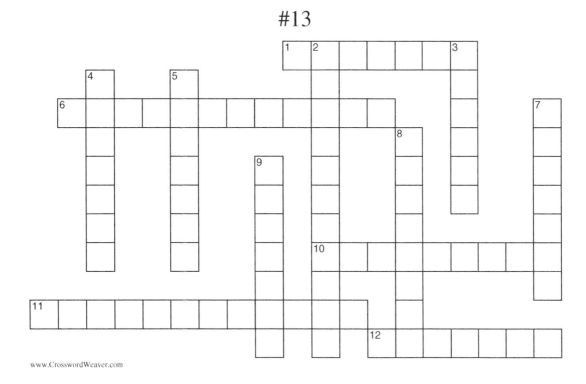

ACROSS

1 not protected by trademark registration
6 inflammation of the lymphatic vessels
10 a system of treating amblyopic by retraining visual habits using guided exercises
11 having an abnormally small head
12 a benign tumor composed of bone tissue

DOWN

2 having a light lean body build
3 the bony apex of the cochlea
4 a cystic tumor of lymphatic origin
5 an individual, organ, or part consisting of tissues of diverse genetic constitution
7 a plaster cast for the trunk and neck
8 any disorder of pregnancy
9 of, or relating to, the tongue

#14

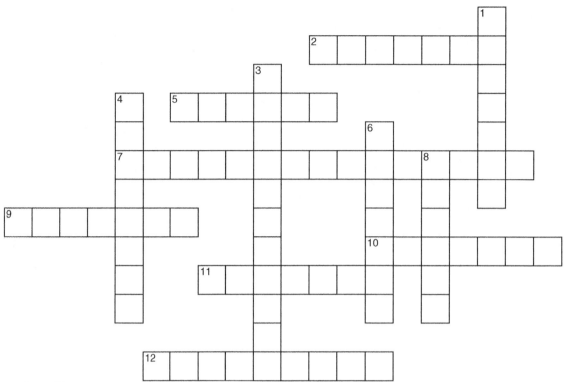

www.CrosswordWeaver.com

ACROSS

2 any fungus of the genus Candida
5 of, relating to, or resembling bone
7 hardening of the kidney
9 free or freed from pathogenic microorganisms
10 incision or division of a muscle
11 a muscle cell
12 the hydrolysis of fat

DOWN

1 a small muscle on each side of the nose that constricts the nasal aperture
3 of or relating to the penis and scrotum
4 alleviating pain or harshness
6 earwax
8 an operation to create an artificial passage for bodily eliminations

#15

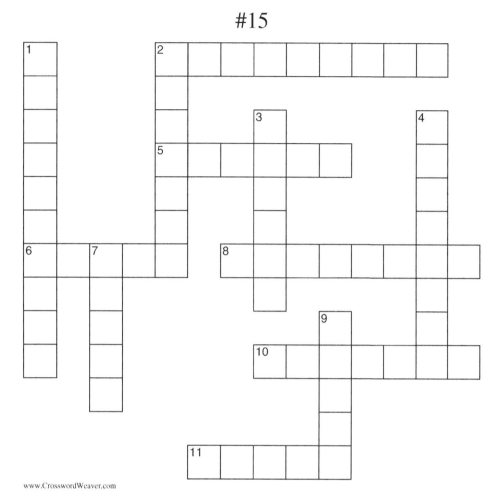

www.CrosswordWeaver.com

ACROSS

2 having the condition of fetid breath

5 a cyst formed under the tongue by obstruction of a gland duct

6 the upper part of the human cranium

8 to diffuse through or penetrate something

10 of, relating to, or situated near the ischium

11 the manual restoration of a displaced body part

DOWN

1 an atypical red blood cell containing iron not bound in hemoglobin

2 a cystic tumor of lymphatic origin

3 throat

4 malignant tumor of the liver

7 any of several diseases characterized by skin lesions

9 a beat or pulsation esp. of the heart

#16

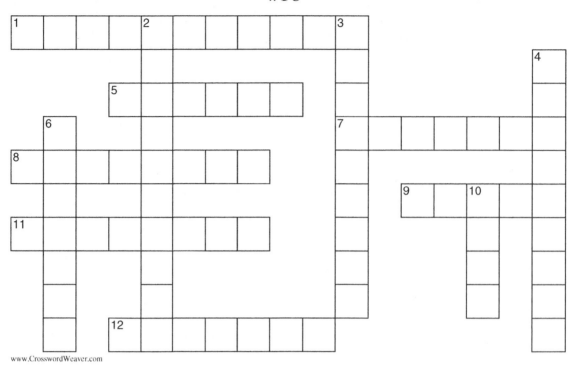

www.CrosswordWeaver.com

ACROSS

1 grafted or transplanted into an abnormal position

5 of or relating to life

7 secreting acid--used esp.of the parietal cells of the gastric glands

8 a disease communicable from animals to humans under natural conditions

9 an elevation in the tempanic membrane of the ear

11 condition in which the total volume of the blood is reduced

12 the back part of the head or skull

DOWN

2 of or relating to the hip and shoulder joints

3 an iron deficiency anemia esp.of adolescent girls that may impart a greenish tint to the skin

4 an exceptionally large red blood cell occuring chiefly in anemias

6 a group of red blood corpuscles resembling a stack of coins

10 an inflammatory swelling of a lymph node esp.in the groin

#17

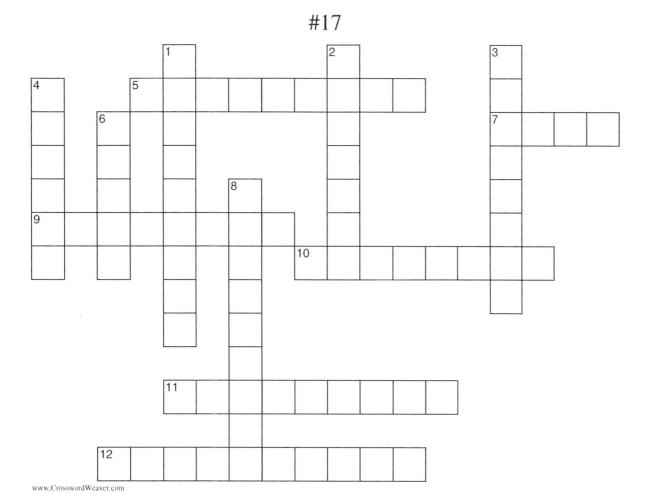

www.CrosswordWeaver.com

ACROSS

5 affected with or characterized by paralysis

7 a brief piercing spasm of pain

9 a disease of the urinary or urogenital organs

10 general physical wasting and malnutrition usu.associated with chronic disease

11 inflammation of a tooth

12 a concretion formed in a lacrimal passage

DOWN

1 a speech defect marked by abnormal repetition of syllables , words, or phrases

2 earache

3 of or relating to the navel

4 big toe

6 a heavy , colorless, and relatively inert gaseous element

8 podiatry

#18

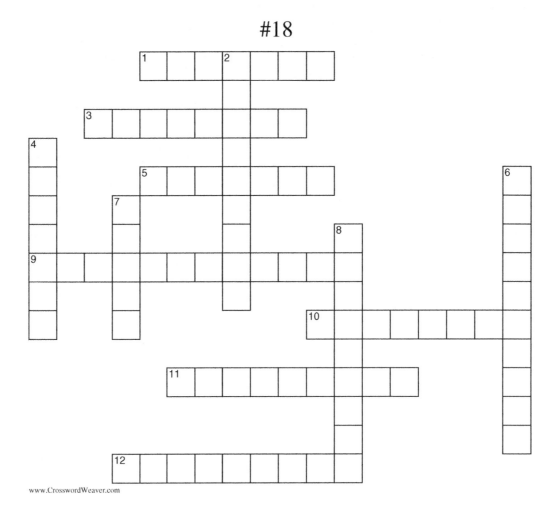

www.CrosswordWeaver.com

ACROSS

1 inflammation of the ilium
3 having small usu. colored spots or drops
5 inflammation of the knee
9 a pathological and commonly congenital enlargement of the tongue
10 the smooth prominance between the eyebrows
11 of, or relating to, or used at the navel
12 a constant usu.burning pain resulting from injury to a peripheral nerve

DOWN

2 the exhausted condition that results from lack of food and water
4 a contracted anatomical part or passage connecting two larger structures or cavities
6 the mesentery uniting the ovary with the body wall
7 a small serous sac between a tendon and a bone
8 a groove between the base of the tongue and the epiglottis

#19

www.CrosswordWeaver.com

ACROSS

1 impaired or decreased tactile sensibility
6 waste material that is secreted by the kidney
7 to wound seriously : mutilate, disable
9 stretched tight : made taut or rigid
10 something that exerts a harmful effect on the body
11 infected with mange

DOWN

1 the indented part of a kidney
2 the production of vocal sounds and esp.speech
3 an agent (as a drug) that increases body tone
4 the last division of the small intestine extending between the jejunum and large intestine
5 to tear in pieces esp.to shred for microscopic examination
8 an involuntary and abnormal contraction of muscle fibers or of a hollow organ that consists largely of involuntary muscle fibers

#20

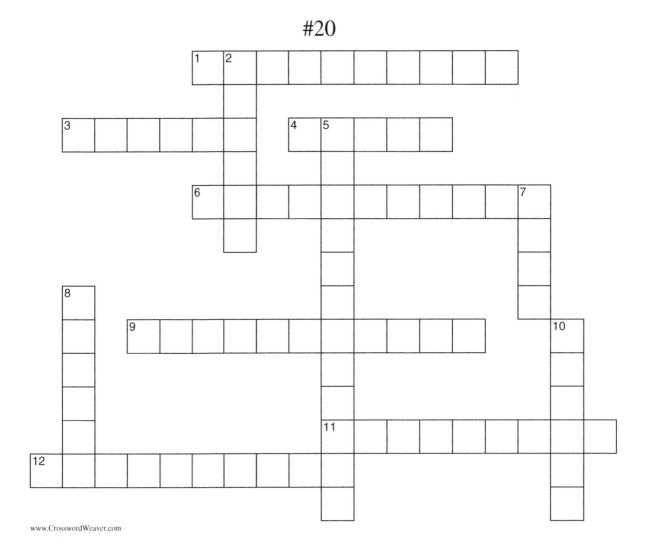

www.CrosswordWeaver.com

ACROSS

1 a concretion formed in a lacrimal passage

3 blackhead

4 to implant (living tissue) surgically

6 finger spelling

9 swelling and protrusion of the blind spot of the eye caused by edema

11 a condition in which the total volume of the blood is reduced

12 an xray of the kidney

DOWN

2 situated opposite to or away from the mouth

5 face lift

7 material stored in an ovum that supplies food to the developing enbyro and cocsists chiefly of proteins, lecithin, and cholesterol

8 suppository

10 inflammatory ringworm of the hair follicles of the beard and scalp usu. accompanied by secondary bacterial infection

#21

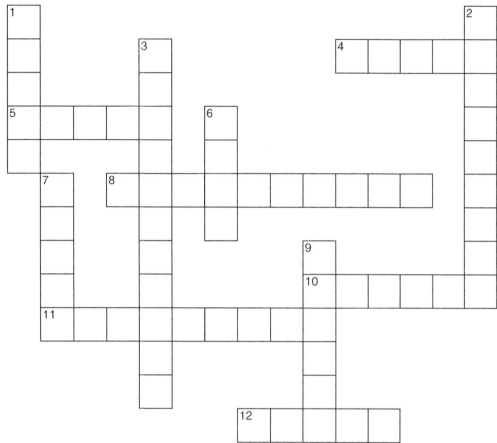

ACROSS

4 wasting accompanying a chronic disease
5 either of the pair of openings of the nose
8 surgical opening of the skull
10 an organism (as a bacterium) that lives only in the presence of oxygen
11 reflecting ultrasound waves
12 a conical vascular body forming the extremity of the penis

DOWN

1 a chronic disease of the nose accompanied by a fetid discharge and marked by atropic changes in the nasal structures
2 to swing backward and forward like a pendulum
3 surgical removal of all or part of the stomach
6 an encircling anatomical structure
7 the semifluid mass of partly digested food expelled by the stomach into the duodenum
9 a small cavity, pit, or discontinuity in an anatomical structure

#22

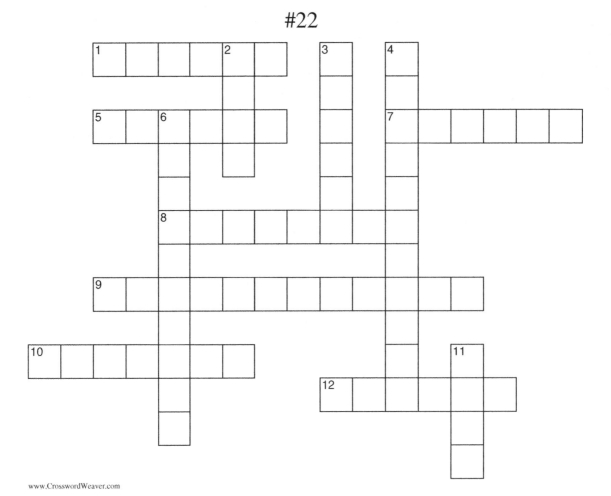

www.CrosswordWeaver.com

ACROSS

1 the condition of being abnormally or exceptionally small in structure
5 an artificial tooth on a dental bridge
7 toward the tail or posterior end
8 a condition characterized by abnormal redness
9 an adenoma of the pituitary gland that is greater than ten millimeters in diameter
10 a tomor that arises from the tissue elements of the thymus
12 of, relating to, or lying in the region of the nape

DOWN

2 the front part of the leg below the knee
3 a pathological paroxysm of activity giving vent to impulse or tension (as in an act of violence)
4 large enough to be observed by the naked eye
6 the surgical excision of part of a nerve
11 the back of the neck

#23

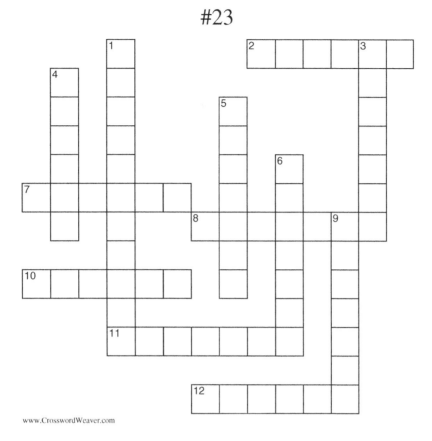

www.CrosswordWeaver.com

ACROSS

2 to remove or destroy esp.by cutting

7 an ancient Chinese discipline involving a continuous series of controlled usu.slow movements designed to improve physical and mental well-being

8 an indefinite feeling of debility or lack of health often indicative of or accompanying the onset of an illness

10 congenital absence of one or more limbs

11 deficiency or absence of bile

12 spread out flat without definite form

DOWN

1 a mental condition and esp. a manic-depressive condition characterized by extreme depression, bodily complaints, and often hallucinations and delusions

3 of, relating to, medicated by, or affecting the sense of touch

4 of or relating to the abdominal cavity

5 curved like a bow

6 earache

9 to flush or spread over or through in the manner of a fluid and esp.blood

#24

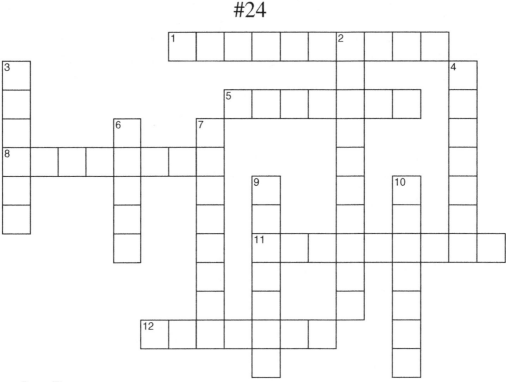

www.CrosswordWeaver.com

ACROSS

1 a surgical operation in which the stomach is sutured to the abdominal wall

5 any fungus of the genus Candida

8 general physical wasting and malnutrition usu.associated with chronic disease

11 of, relating to, or involving a nerve root

12 masturbation

DOWN

2 a calculus in a vein usu.resulting from the calcification of an old thrombus

3 having an adhesive quality

4 a painful condition of the big toe caused by gout

6 a congenital or acquired usu.highly pigmented area of the skin that is either flat or raised:mole

7 a fatty irregular yellow patch or nodule on the skin that is associated esp.with disturbance of cholesterol metabolism

9 abnormal dryness of a body part or tissue (as the skin)

10 a tumor or mass growing from a nerve and usu.consisting of nerve fibers

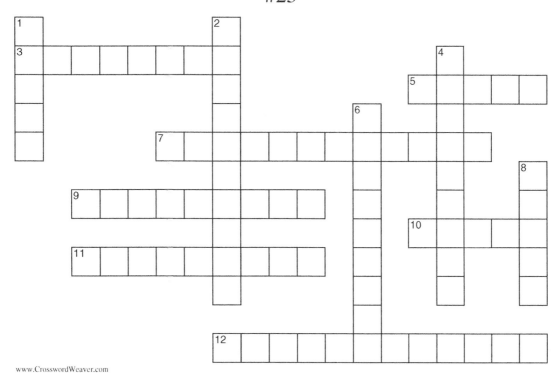

ACROSS

3 to cause to lose flesh so as to become very thin

5 of, relating to, or produced by the blood or the circulation of the blood

7 of or relating to the lips and the tongue

9 gliding joint

10 the indented part of the kidney

11 inflammation of the glans penis

12 the presence of excess lactic acid in the blood

DOWN

1 oxidation-reduction

2 a chemical compound (as a drug or pesticide) that is foreign to a living organism

4 a thin membrane that gives support to cappillaries surrounding the tubule of a nephron

6 living, active, or occurring in the absence of free oxygen

8 the posterior more or less vertical part of the lower jaw on each side which articulates with the skull

#26

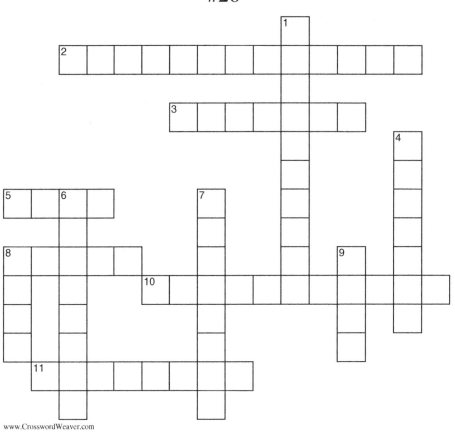

www.CrosswordWeaver.com

ACROSS

2 a dry thickened lusterless condition of the eyeball resulting esp.from a severe deficiency of vitamin A

3 the habit of unconsciously gritting or grinding the teeth esp.in situations of stress or during sleep

5 a circle of light appearing to surround a luminous body; esp: one seen as the result of the presence of glaucoma

8 of, relating to, or produced by the blood or the circulation of blood

10 involving or relating to many bones

11 a scar resulting from formation and contraction of fibrous tissue in a flesh wound

DOWN

1 excretion of potassium in the urine esp.in excessive amounts

4 inflammation of the matrix of a nail often leading to suppuration and loss of the nail

6 of, relating to, or being the suture shaped like the Greek letter lambda that connects the occipital and parietal bones

7 the presence of excess bile in the blood usu. indicative of liver disease

8 a short dry cough

9 a metabolic disease marked by painful inflammation of the joints, deposits of urates in and around the joints, and usually an excessive amount of uric acid in the blood

#27

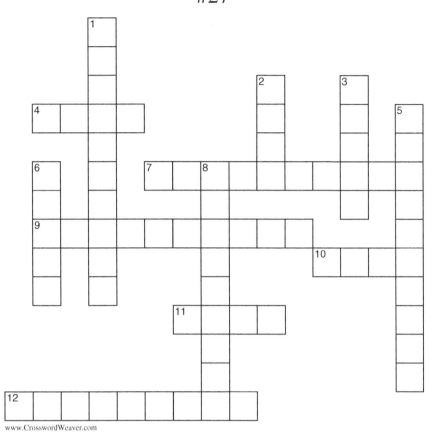

www.CrosswordWeaver.com

ACROSS

4 the serum or watery part of milk that is separated from the coagulable part or curd, is rich in lactose, minerals, and vitamins, and contains lactalbumin and traces of fat

7 of, relating to, affecting, or being the region of the joint between the sacrum and the ilium

9 freeze dry

10 a broad mass of chiefly transverse nerve fibers in the mammalian brain stem lying ventral to the cerebellum at the anterior end of the medulla oblangata

11 of, relating to, or located in the region of the ear

12 the surgical formation of an opening into the cecum to serve as an artificial anus

DOWN

1 surgical incision into the rumen

2 an elevation in the tempanic membrane of the ear

3 an attack of acute abdominal pain localized in a hollow organ and often caused by spasm, obstruction or twisting

5 gigantism

6 of or relating to the cheek, the side of the head, or the zygomatic bone

8 milk secreted for a few days after parturition and characterized by high protein and antibody content

#28

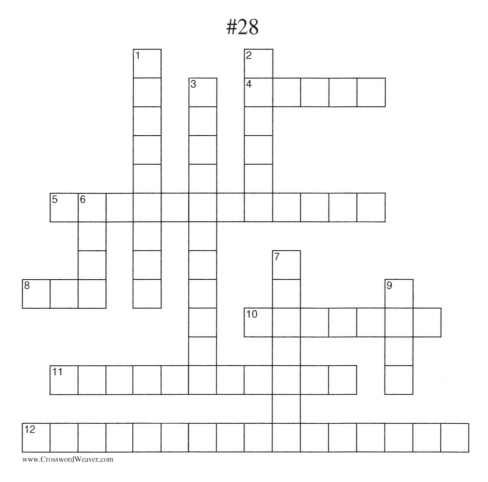

www.CrosswordWeaver.com

ACROSS

4 irritatingly sharp and harsh or unpleasantly pungent in taste or odor

5 a delusion that one has become or has assumed the characteristics of a wolf

8 an abnormal growth or a cyst protruding from a surface esp.of the skin

10 a noncaloric fat substitute that consists of sucrose esters resistant to absorption by the digestive system due to their large size

11 producing swelling

12 persistent decrease in the number of blood platelets that is often associated with hemorrhagic conditions

DOWN

1 nosebleed

2 deficiency of color esp.of the face

3 subnormal temperature of the body

6 an opening of the mouth wide while taking a deep breath often as an involuntary reaction to fatique or boredom

7 a usual liquid substance capable of dissolving or dispersing one or more other substances

9 tempanic membrane

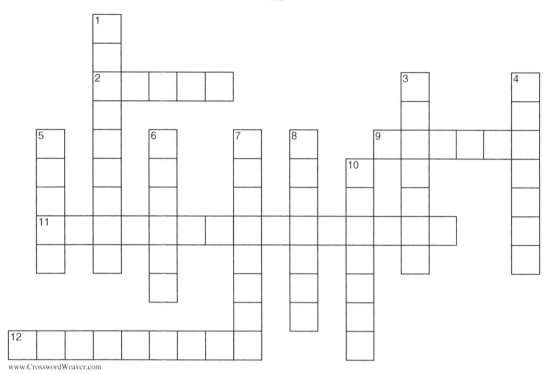

www.CrosswordWeaver.com

ACROSS

2 a viscid slippery secretion that is usu.rich in mucins and is produced by mucous membranes which it moistens and protects

9 a vascular tissue causing a superficial opacity of the cornea and occuring esp.in trachoma

11 hardening of the kidney

12 an especially congenital absence of teeth

DOWN

1 a device which graphically records motion or pressure (as of blood)

3 pain in one or more muscles

4 a rose-shaped cluster of cells

5 the part of the leg between the knee and the ankle in humans or a corrisponding part in other vertebrates

6 an offspring of two animals or plants of different races, breeds, varieties, species, or genera

7 the presence of glucose in the blood

8 a serious eating disorder that occurs chiefly in females, is characterized by compulsive overeating usually followed by self-induced vomiting or laxative or diuretic abuse, and is often accompanied by guilt and depression

10 a lustrous ductile mettalic element

#30

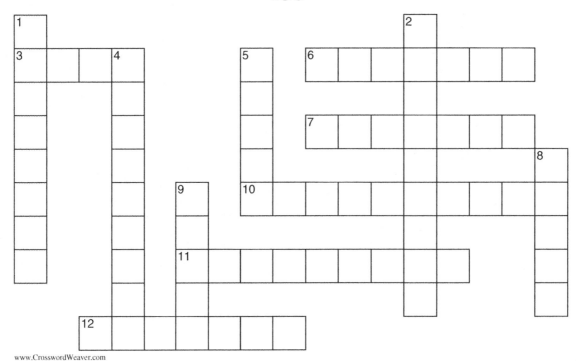

www.CrosswordWeaver.com

ACROSS

3 a pathological swelling or enlargement (as of a rheumatic joint)

6 a vascular membrane containing large branched pigment cells that lies between the retina and sclera of the eye

7 earwax

10 a granulocyte that is the chief phagocytic white blood cell

11 reflecting ultrasound waves

12 any of various sulfer-containing fibrous proteins that form the chemical basis of horny epidermal tissues (as hair and nails)

DOWN

1 rich in oil or fat

2 atropy and shriveling of the skin or mucous membrane esp.of the vulva where it is often a precancerous lesion

4 a recovering of consciousness (as from anesthesia)

5 a fold or mucous membrane partly or wholly closing the orifice of the vagina

8 a chronic inflammation (as gonorrhea) of a bodily orifice usu.accompanied by an abnormal discharge

9 an enveloping case or sheath of an anatomical part

#31

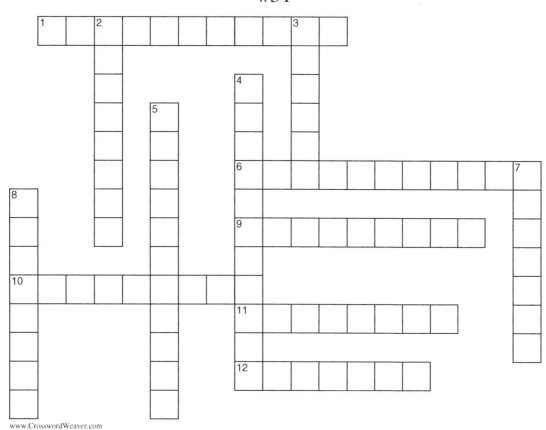

www.CrosswordWeaver.com

ACROSS

1 the presence of an excess of carbon dioxide in the blood
6 an anatomical malformation
9 of, relating to, being, or lying in the region of the inferior part of the sphenoid bone
10 murder of a mother by her son or daughter
11 the presence of glucose in the blood
12 a condition of lack of development of intellectual capacity

DOWN

2 of, relating to, or occurring in or on the chest
3 inflammation of the iris of the eye
4 paralysis of the sphincter of the iris
5 impairment of mathmatical ability due to an organic condition of the brain
7 a mold of a lesion or defect used as a guide in applying medical treatment (as in radiotherapy) or in performing reconstruction surgery esp.on the face
8 lead poisoning

#32

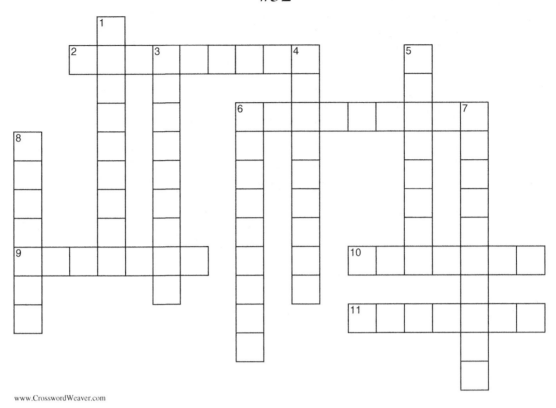

www.CrosswordWeaver.com

ACROSS

2 a foot deformity characterized by an abnormally high arch
6 the operation of suturing the end of a tendon to a bone
9 secreting acid--used esp.of the parietal cells of the gastric glands
10 a cutaneous eruption marked by large flat pustules that have a hardened base surrounded by inflammation and occur esp.on lower legs
11 of or derived from swine

DOWN

1 a condition in which a tooth or the jaw is posterior to its proper occlusal position
3 inflammation of a crypt (as an anal crypt)
4 having two or more digits wholly or partly united
5 producing or tending to produce blisters
6 a gene that is taken from the genome of one organism and introduced into the genome of another organism by artificial techniques
7 a toxic condition produced by excessive intake of salicytic acid or salicylates and marked by ringing in the ears, nausea, and vomiting
8 an individual or fetus abnormal in having a single eye or the usual two orbits fused

#33

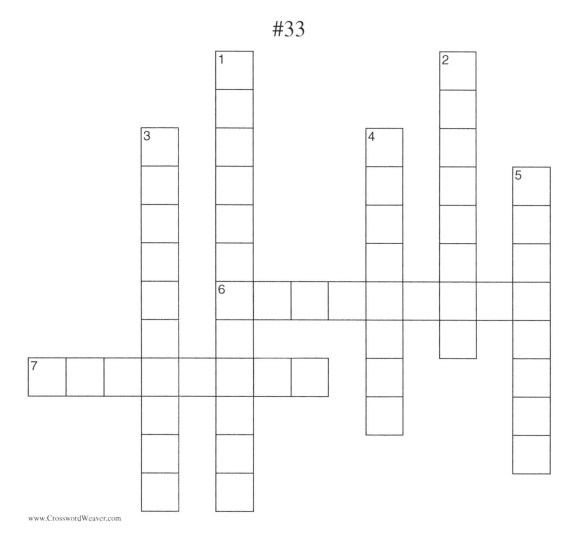

ACROSS

6 the closure or blockage (as of a wound) by or as if by a tampon esp.to stop bleeding

7 inflammation of the vitreous body of the eye

DOWN

1 a crust or hard coating

2 of or relating to tears

3 toothache

4 inducing contraction of uterine smooth muscle

5 an acute contagious staplococcal or streptococcal skin disease characterized by vesicles, pustules, and yellowish crusts

#34

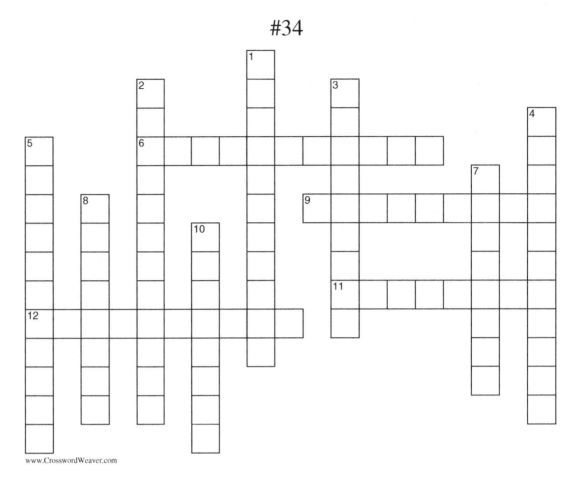

www.CrosswordWeaver.com

ACROSS

6 a green pigment that occurs in bile and is formed by breakdown of hemoglobin

9 the closure or blockage (as of a wound) by or as if by a tampon esp.to stop bleeding

11 an acute contagious staphlococcal or streptococcal skin disease characterized by vesicles, pustules, and yellowish crusts

12 toothache

DOWN

1 the apparent production of motion in objects (as by a spiritualistic medium) without contact or other physical means

2 a crust or hard coating

3 sexual excitement associated with urine or with urination

4 situated or extending between the ribs

5 the description or study of the phenomena of death and of psychological mechanisms for coping with them

7 of or relating to tears

8 inducing contraction of uterine smooth muscle

10 inflammation of the vitreous body of the eye

#35

ACROSS

2 of or relating to the hip and shoulder joints

4 a terminal patient whose brain is nonfunctional and the rest of whose body can be kept functioning only by the extensive use of mechanical devices and nutrient solutions (term is usu.used derisively)

7 exaggerated backward curvature of the thoracic region of the spinal column

8 any of various small surgical instruments with a shape resembling that of a spade

10 a virus or living organism capable of causing a communicable disease

11 beginning to come into being or to become apparent

12 to remove (absorbed material) from an absorbant by means of a solvent

DOWN

1 exaggerated forward curvature of the lumbar and cervical regions of the spinal column

3 any of several emulsifiers used in the preparation of some pharmaceuticals

5 a substance that corrodes

6 a small circumscribed elevation of the skin containing pus and having an inflamed base

9 an eruption occurring esp.in tertiary syphilis consisting of vesicles having an inflamed base and filled with serous purulent or bloody fluid which dries up and forms large blackish conical crusts

www.CrosswordWeaver.com

#36

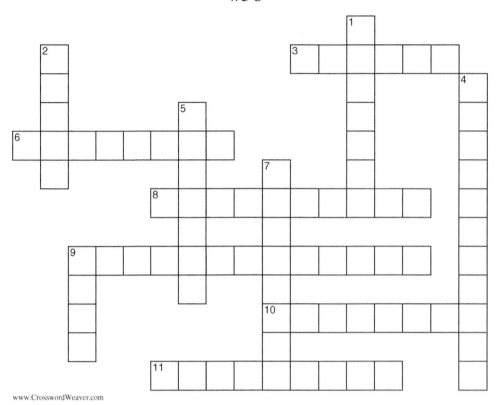

www.CrosswordWeaver.com

ACROSS

3 an elongated depression of the ear that separates the helix and antihelix

6 a diagram outlining the behavioral or medical history of a family's members over several generations

8 a condition in which the proper meaning of words cannot be remembered

9 infestation with a disease caused by parasitic worms

10 abnormal drowsiness

11 a sexual perversion characterized by pleasure in being subjected to pain or humiliation esp.by a love object

DOWN

1 slight or partial paralysis

2 a chronic problem patient who does not respond to treatment (med.slang usually disparaging)

4 a hemoglobin-containing fragment of a red blood cell

5 a neurotransmitter that plays a role in regulating various physiological functions (as contraction of gastrointestinal muscle and inhibition of insulin)

7 of or relating to the navel

9 an enveloping case or sheath of an anatomical part

#37

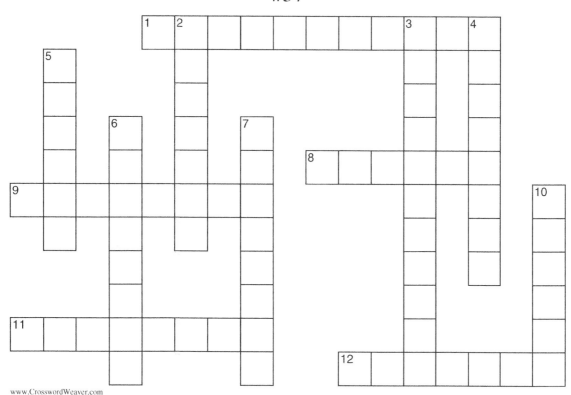

www.CrosswordWeaver.com

ACROSS

1 an overlapping esp.of successive layers of tissue in the surgical closure of a wound
8 environment
9 dislocation of an anatomical part
11 prolonged and usu.abnormal inability to obtain adequate sleep
12 having a structure like that of a feather esp:being a muscle in which fibers extend obliquely from either side of a central tendon

DOWN

2 infection with or disease caused by a fungus
3 the drawing of air into the lungs
4 urination at night esp.when excessive
5 wrist
6 the midpoint of the lower border of the human mandible
7 one billionth of a gram
10 suppository

#38

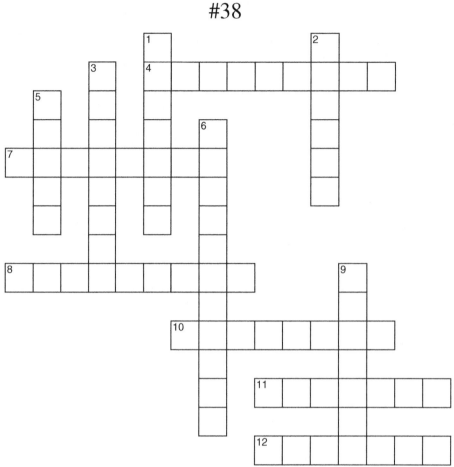

ACROSS

4 of, relating to, or connecting muscles and nerves

7 inflammation of the vulva

8 act or process of combining or treating with water

10 one that practices anal intercourse esp. with a boy as a passive partner

11 the quality or state of being fed or gratified to or beyond capacity

12 presence of anexcess of fat or lipids in the blood

DOWN

1 the absence or underdevelopment of the mammary glands

2 deposit of small calculous concretions in the kidneys and urinary bladder

3 a small valve or fold

5 to expel air from the lungs suddenly with a sharp short noise

6 originating in the mind or in mental or emotional conflict

9 to inhale and exhale air successively

#39

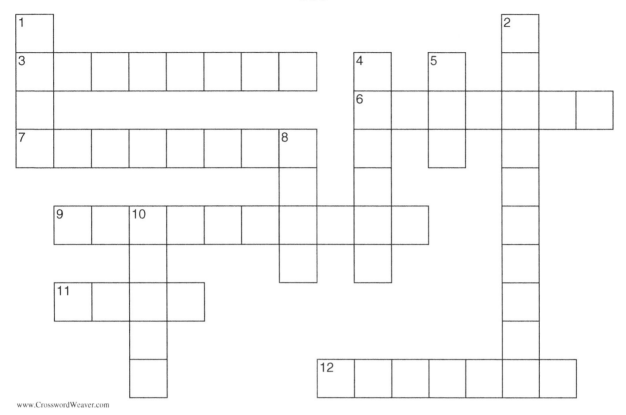

www.CrosswordWeaver.com

ACROSS

3 attraction toward a particular object or in a specific direction

6 to combine with oxygen

7 a condition characterized by abnormal redness

9 a plasma protein produced in the liver in the presence of vitamin k and converted into thrombin by the action of various activators (as thromboplastin) in the clotting of blood

11 a small blister

12 a crescent-shaped body part

DOWN

1 a bony outgrowth

2 excessive secretion from the nose

4 an artificial tooth on a dental bridge

5 local and habitual spasmodic motion of particular muscles esp.of the face

8 a circumscribed surface lesion of disease (as measles)

10 oil

#40

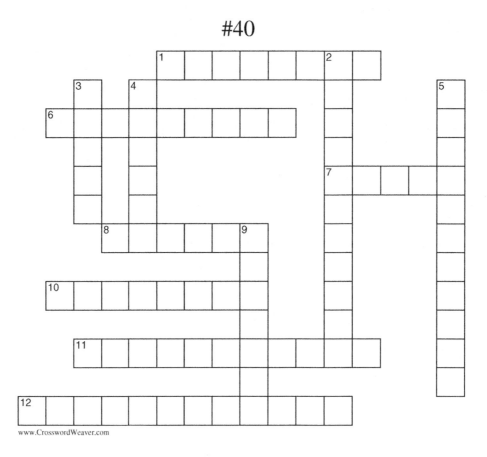

www.CrosswordWeaver.com

ACROSS

1 lesbian
6 a spindle-shaped cell of fibrous tissue
7 low spirits:melancholy
8 not manifest or detectable by clinical methods alone
10 the practice of freezing the body of a person who has died from a disease in hopes of restoring life at some future time when a cure for the disease has been developed
11 characterized by, allowing, or being a backward flow (as of blood)
12 an abnormal deficiency of iron in the blood

DOWN

2 a method of removing tattoos from skin in which moist gauze pads saturated with sodium chloride are used to abrade the tattooed area by rubbing
3 an object resembling a penis used for sexual stimulation
4 of, devoted to, or tending to arouse sexual desire
5 profuse and often emotionally charged speech that mimics coherent speech but is usu.unintelligible to the listener and that is uttered in some states of religious ecstacy and in some schizophrenic states
9 of, relating to, or involved in coughing

#41

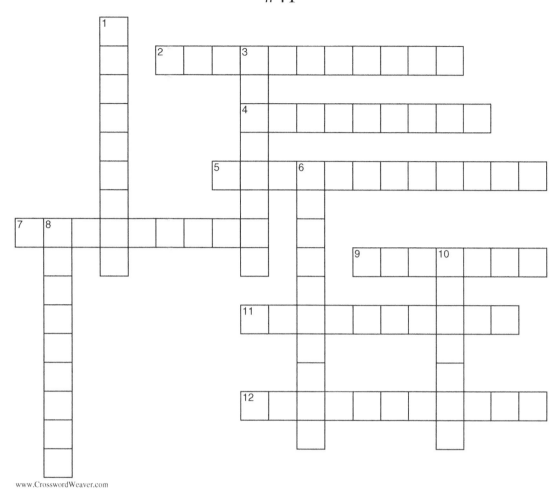

www.CrosswordWeaver.com

ACROSS

2 elevation of the line of vision of one eye above that of the other: upward strabismus
4 inflammation of a tooth
5 face lift
7 a state or period during which the symptoms of a disease are abated
9 food; esp.a suspension or solution of nutrients in a state suitable for absorption
11 toothless
12 characterized by piercing or stabbing sensations

DOWN

1 relating to or influencing the force of muscular contraction
3 a modification of the voice resembling bleating heard on auscultation of the chest in some diseases (as in pleurisy with effusion)
6 percussion
8 hard and dense like ivory
10 urinary calculus

#42

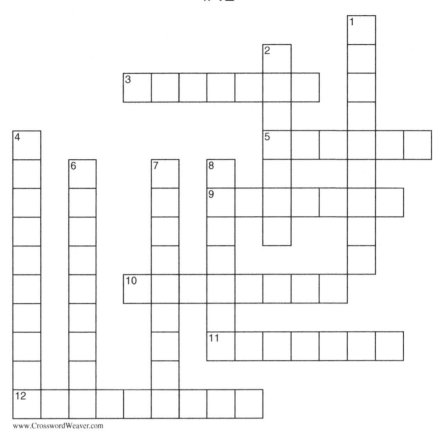

www.CrosswordWeaver.com

ACROSS

3 synovial fluid
5 the final period in the normal life span
9 to divide (as a solution) into equal parts
10 a new growth of tissue serving no physiological function : tumor
11 a small collapsible tube fitted with a hypodermic needle for injecting a single dose of a medicinal agent
12 to grind, crush, and chew (food) with or as if with the teeth in preparation for swallowing

DOWN

1 caused by parasitic worms
2 resembling a dilated tortuous vein
4 love of or sexual desire for one's own body
6 infestation with or disease caused by tapeworms
7 of, relating to, or invested with mental or emotional energy
8 clubfoot

#43

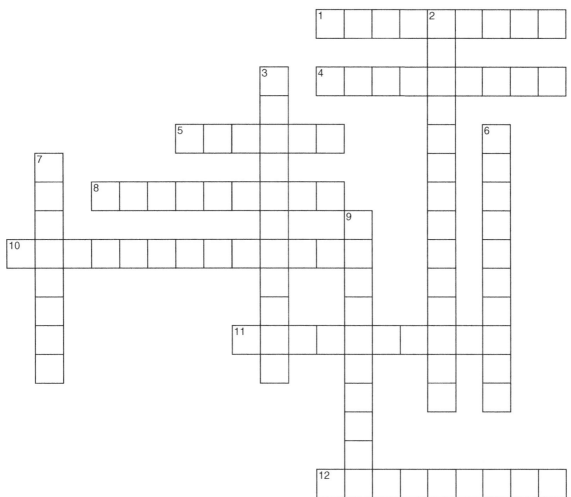

ACROSS

1 surgical removal of all or part of a bone
4 surgical incision of the urinary bladder
5 a fibrous ring of cartilage attached to the rim of a joint
8 to supply with nerves
10 surgical excision of a fallopian tube
11 any of several diseases usu. of hereditary origin characterized by rough, thick, and scaly skin
12 the operation of suturing the end of a tendon to a bone

DOWN

2 production of gallstones
3 a branch of medicine that deals with the problems and diseases of old age and aging people
6 expectoration of blood from some part of the respiratory tract
7 infantile speech whether in infants or in older speakers (as from mental retardation)
9 freeze-dry

#44

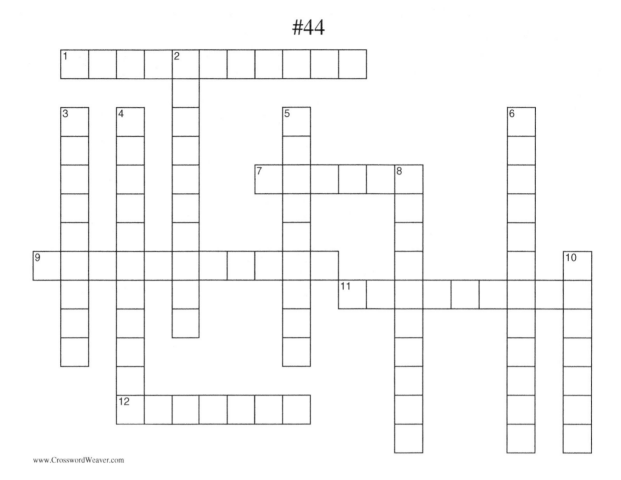

www.CrosswordWeaver.com

ACROSS

1 a disorganized form of schizophrenia characterized esp.by incoherence, delusions lacking an underlying theme, and affect that is flat, inappropriate, or silly

7 a gluey protein substance esp.of wheat flour that causes dough to be sticky

9 sleep of excessive depth or duration

11 a drug that promotes the enhancement of cognition and memory and the facilitation of learning

12 the place at which a nervous impulse passes from one neuron to another

DOWN

2 hay fever

3 the shaft of a long bone

4 formation of fat in the living body esp. when excessive or abnormal

5 inflammation of a vein

6 plastic surgery of the penis or scrotum

8 a condition characterized by brief attacks of sleep often occurring with cataplexy and hypnagogic hallucinations

10 an abnormal congenital or acquired position of an organ or part

#45

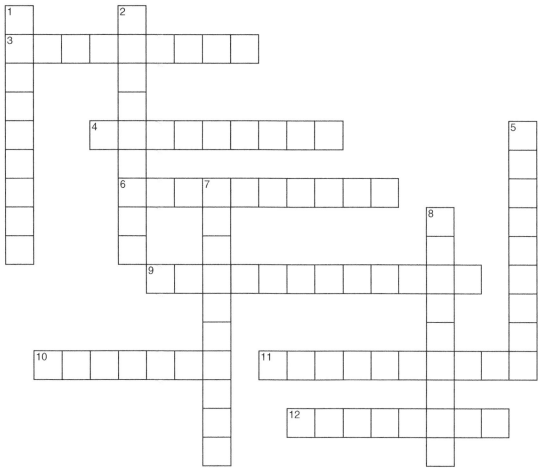

www.CrosswordWeaver.com

ACROSS

3 a toxic condition caused by the extravasation of urine into bodily tissues

4 a constant usu. burning pain resulting from injury to a peripheral nerve

6 scientific study of hair and its diseases

9 a surgical puncture of a cavity of the body (as with a trocar or aspirator) usu.to draw off any abnormal effusion

10 loss or impairment of the sense of smell

11 surgical excision of the uvula

12 the presence of fungi in the blood

DOWN

1 of, relating to, occurring in, or lying in the region of the external genital organs

2 any of various surgical instruments for holding tissues away from the field of operation

5 pregnancy

7 a muscle that contracts the skin into wrinkles esp: one that draws the eyebrows together and wrinkles the brow in frowning

8 surgical incision of the nose

#46

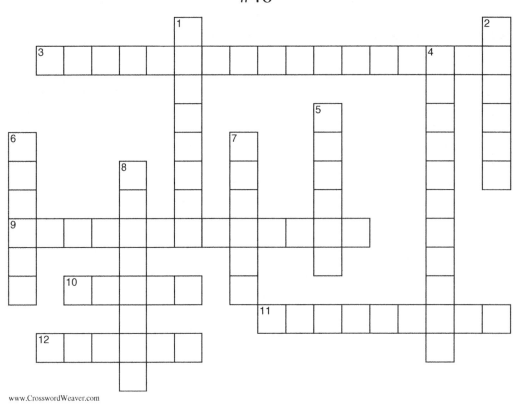

www.CrosswordWeaver.com

ACROSS

3 a benign epithelial tumor developing from the hair follicles esp.on the face

9 inflammation of both spinal cord and nerves

10 a chronic inflammation (as gonorrhea) of a bodily orifice usu.accompanied by an abnormal discharge

11 a word coined by a psychotic individual that is meaningless except to the coiner

12 an inflamed swelling of the small fluid-filled sac of the first joint of the big toe accompanied by enlargement and protrusion of the joint

DOWN

1 surgical severance of nerve fibers connecting the frontal lobes to the thalamus for relief of some mental disorders

2 a sharp-pointed and commonly two-edged surgical instrument used to make small incisions

4 forming or capable of forming teeth

5 of a kind that is likely to be undertaken only to save life

6 a flat surface of bone esp.of the skull

7 the innermost digit of the foot : big toe

8 the presence of excess bile inthe blood usu. indicative of liver disease

#47

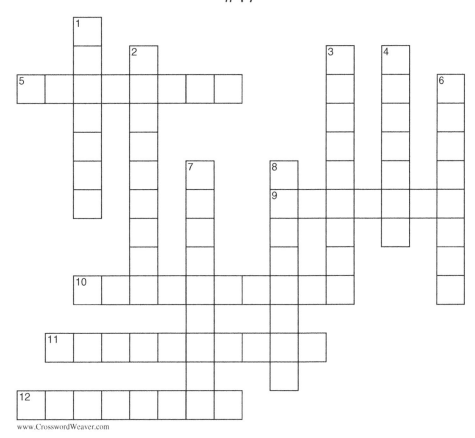

www.CrosswordWeaver.com

ACROSS

5 notched or toothed on the edge
9 dislocation of an anatomical part
10 a condition characterized by abnormally small and imperfectly developed extremities
11 to make involuntary stops and repititions in speaking
12 a discharge of pus

DOWN

1 abnormal dryness of a body part or tissue (as the skin)
2 facilitating the urinary excretion of salt and esp.of sodium ion
3 an irresistable impulse to start fires
4 a small muscle on each side of the nose that constricts the nasal aperture
6 the study of the general principles of scientific classification
7 herniation of the rectum through a defect in the intervening fascia into the vagina
8 containing, consisting of, or being pus

#48

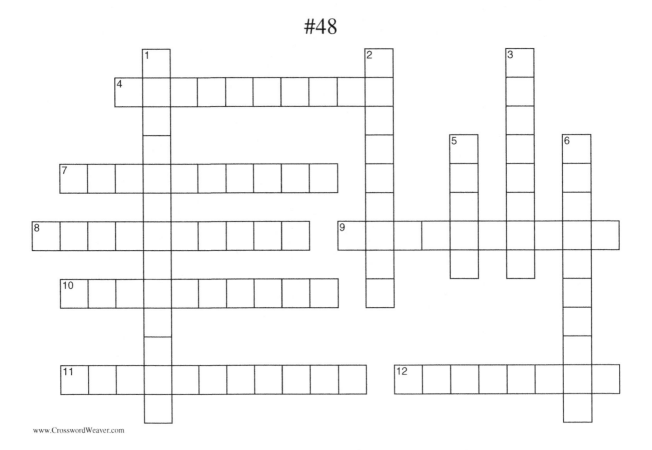

ACROSS

4 the effusion of blood into a body cavity (as the scrotum)

7 relating to or being the ankle joint

8 a simple stereoscope used in the study of depth perception

9 seizure

10 giantism

11 cystostomy

12 a minute reddish or purplish spot containing blood that appears in skin or mucous membrane as a result of localized hemorrage

DOWN

1 having an affinity for neurons

2 surgical incision of the abdomen

3 having or growing in a form like that of a cluster of grapes

5 a knoblike protuberance (as of a bone or muscle)

6 union of two or more separate bones to form a simple bone

#49

www.CrosswordWeaver.com

ACROSS

4 a flash of light produced in a phosphorescent substance by an ionizing event

5 a bodily structure lying near or associated with another (as a vein accompanying an artery)

7 a suspension of a large amount of precipitated material (as in milk of magnesia) in a small volume of a watery vehicle

8 image

10 spread out flat without definite form

12 pain in the stomach or epigastrum esp.of a neuralgic type

DOWN

1 of, relating to, being, or performed by intubation of the stomach by way of the nasal passages

2 of or relating to the buttocks or the gluteal muscles

3 a surgical operation in which the stomach is sutured to the abdominal wall

6 having, showing, or characterized by an ability to think clearly and rationally

9 the inward curved rim of the external ear

11 the pendant fleshy lobe in the middle of the posterior border of the soft palate

#50

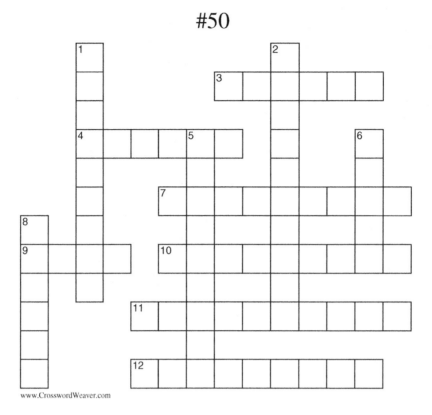

www.CrosswordWeaver.com

ACROSS

3 to make thinner or more liquid by admixture

4 an unfilled space within a mass

7 a backward displacement; spec: a condition in which a tooth or the jaw is posterior to its proper occlusal position

9 a device used to arrest bleeding from vessels or tissue during operations

10 movement of a tooth out of its normal position esp. as a result of periodontal disease

11 not produced by natural means

12 a torn and ragged wound

DOWN

1 of, relating to, or characterized by the direction of love toward an object (as the mother) that satifies nonsexual needs (as hunger)

2 made up of loosely aggregated particles

5 the beginning of breast development at the onset of puberty

6 the topmost part of the skull or head

8 not manifest or detectable by clinical methods alone

#51

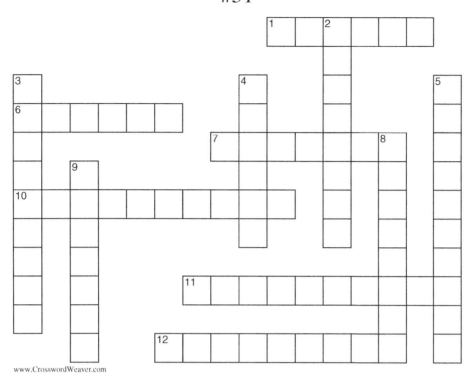

www.CrosswordWeaver.com

ACROSS

1 a small anatomical prominance or projection
6 the substance of the spinal cord
7 an elongated particle (as in a sicle cell) that appears as a spindle-shaped body under a polarizing microscope
10 inflammation of the gums that is often accompanied by tenderness or bleeding
11 a toxin (as ricin) produced by a plant
12 a congenital abnormality (as total or partial absence) affecting only the distal half of a limb

DOWN

2 of, caused by, or infected by leprosy
3 a recovering of consciousness (as from anesthesia)
4 a substance that is in the blood of individuals with syphilis and is responsible for positive serological reactions for syphilis
5 pain in one side of the head
8 a variable often familial learning disability involving difficulties in acquiring and processing language that is typically manifested by a lack of proficiency in reading, spelling, and writing
9 to receive from a parent or ancestor by genetic transmission

#52

ACROSS

2 a patch of skin that is altered in color but usu. not elevated

6 a small mass of rounded or irregular shape: as a small abnormal knobby bodily protuberance (as a tumerous growth or a calcification near an arthritic joint)

8 excitement of psychotic proportions manifested by mental and physical hyperactivity, disorganization of behavior, and elevation of mood

11 an enveloping membrane or layer of body tissue

12 a process of disintegration or dissolution (as of cells)

DOWN

1 an extremely toxic chemical warfare agent

3 a place or site of an event, activity or thing

4 a watery discharge from the mucous membrane esp. of the eyes or nose

5 winding or coiled around: convoluted

7 reduced excretion of urine

9 buttocks

10 a woman experienced in childbirth who provides advice, information, emotional support, and physical comfort to a mother before, during, and just after childbirth

#53

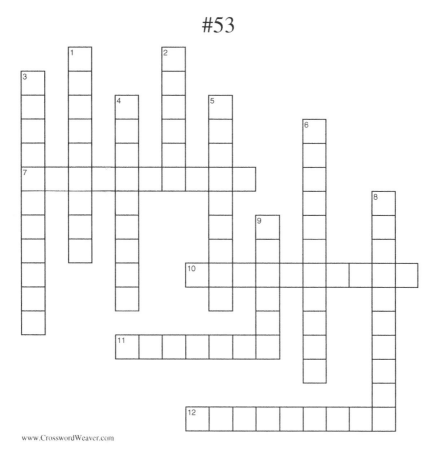

www.CrosswordWeaver.com

ACROSS

7 moving or tending to move the eyeball
10 an atypical red blood cell all containing iron not bound in hemoglobin
11 to close up or block off: obstruct
12 atropy and shriveling of the skin or mucous membranes esp.of the vulva where it is often a precancerois lesion

DOWN

1 falling off or shed at a certain stage in the life cycle
2 a dense cottony or downy growth specif: the soft downy hair that covers the fetus
3 a morbid fear of water
4 a condition marked by an abnormal increase of ketone bodies in the circulating blood
5 pain resulting from a stimulous (as a light touch of the skin) which would not normally provoke pain
6 a hemoglobin-containing fragment of a red blood celll
8 the recurrance of stenosis in a blood vessel or heart valve following apparently successful trearment (as by balloon angioplasty)
9 an enzyme that catalyzes the hydrolysis of urea into ammonia and carbon dioxide

#54

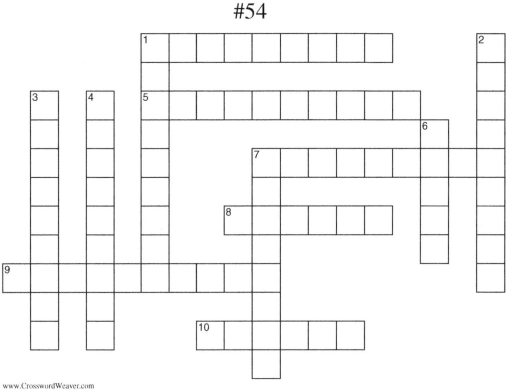

www.CrosswordWeaver.com

ACROSS

1 a constant usu. burning pain resulting from injury to a peripheral nerve
5 having an affinity for cells
7 not accompanied or characterized by jaundice
8 the active phase of the hair growth cycle preceding telogen
9 one who hates women
10 the cavity beneath the junction of the arm or anterior appendage and shoulder or pectoral girdle containing the axillary artery and vein, a part of the brachial plexus of nerves, many lymph nodes, and fat and areolar tissue; esp: armpit

DOWN

1 the surgical formation of an opening into the cecum to serve as an artificial anus
2 lack or loss of the ability to perform simple arithmetic tasks
3 the process of the malleus of the ear
4 surgical excision of selected portions of the frontal cortex of the brain esp: for the relief of medically intractable epilepsy
6 any of several generally abnormal sounds heard on auscultation
7 the congenital complete or partial absence of one or both jaws

#55

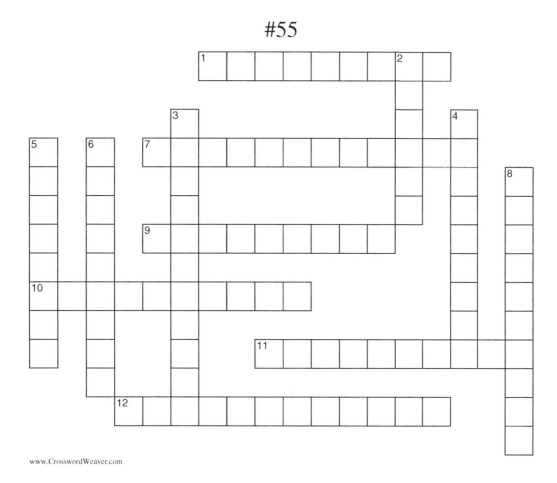

www.CrosswordWeaver.com

ACROSS

1 a woman whomhas never borne a child
7 a condition in which the spermatozoa in seminal fluid are dead or motionless
9 Down Syndrome
10 the part of the pharynx that is below the soft palate and above the epiglottis and is continuous with the mouth
11 an improper or incomplete descent of a testis into the scrotum
12 a congenital abnormality (as spina bifida) characterized by a cleft of the spinal column

DOWN

2 an instrument used in dentistry to enlarge and clean out a root canal
3 tending to attract leucocytes
4 to beat rapidly, irregulary, or forcibly--used esp.of the heart
5 a tendency on part of an individual or group toward excessive or irrational suspiciousness and distrustfulness of others
6 the condition of having papular lesions
8 surgical incision of a kidney (as for the extraction of a calculus)

#56

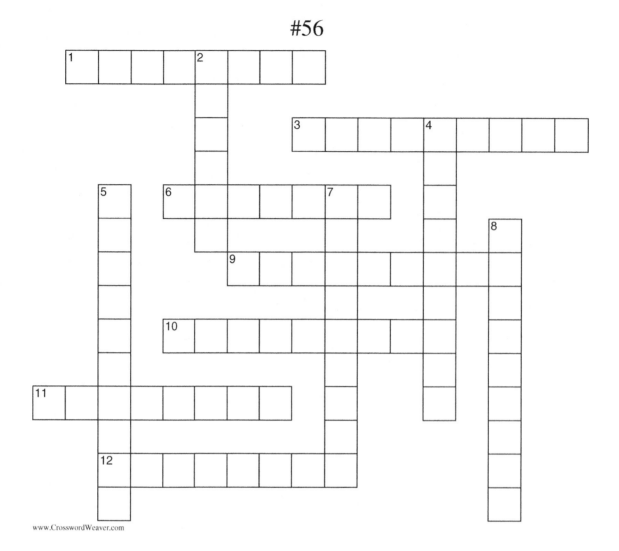

www.CrosswordWeaver.com

ACROSS

1 suggesting a kidney in outline
3 occurring in the normal place
6 likely to cause injury
9 chicken pox
10 infestation with or disease caused by tapeworm
11 spread widely apart : wide open or distended
12 an undifferentiated cell capable of giving rise to muscle cells

DOWN

2 a deep wrinkle
4 inhibition of uterine contraction
5 the surgical excision of part of a nerve
7 a chromosome that lacks a synaptic mate
8 the secretion and yielding of milk by the mammary gland

#57

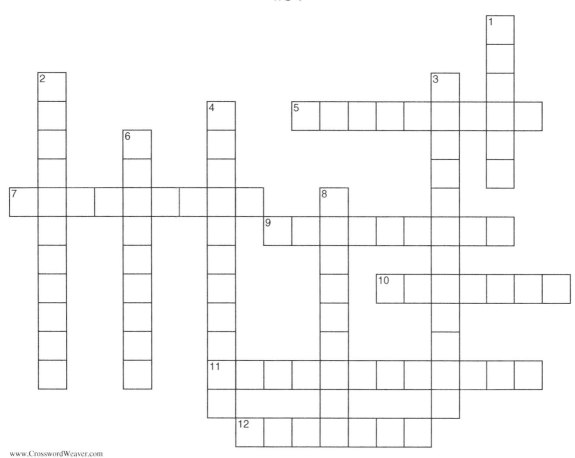

www.CrosswordWeaver.com

ACROSS

5 nosebleed
7 white blood cell
9 covered with warty elevations
10 an abnormal and constant craving for food
11 surgical excision of the navel
12 a movement that lacks directional orientation and depends upon the intensity of stimulation

DOWN

1 any of the folds of the margin of the vulva
2 of, relating to, or being feelings of persecution : paranoid
3 plastic surgery of the vagina
4 severe and intractable constipation
6 gallstone
8 to pulverize thoroughly by rubbing or grinding

#58

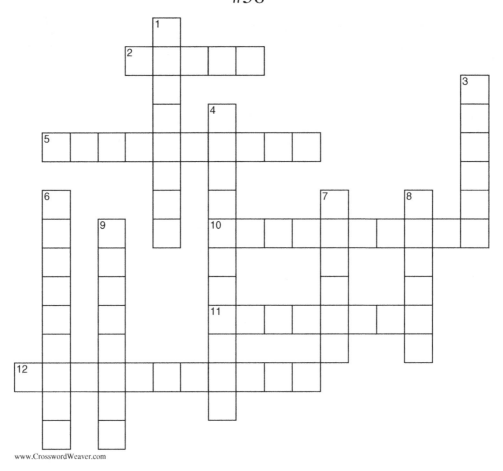

www.CrosswordWeaver.com

ACROSS

2 the last division of the small intestine extending between the jejunum and large intestine
5 difficulty in articulating words due to disease of the central nervous system--compare Dysphasia
10 pain in the breast -- called also mastalgia
11 presence of bile in the urine
12 the surgical removal of a portion of the skull

DOWN

1 having or being a smooth hairless surface
3 a cyst formed under the tongue by obstruction of a gland duct
4 platelet
6 any of a genus of kelps of which some have been used to dilate the cervix in performing an abortion
7 back; esp: the entire dorsal surface of an animal
8 of or relating to a fingernail or toenail
9 chlamydia

#59

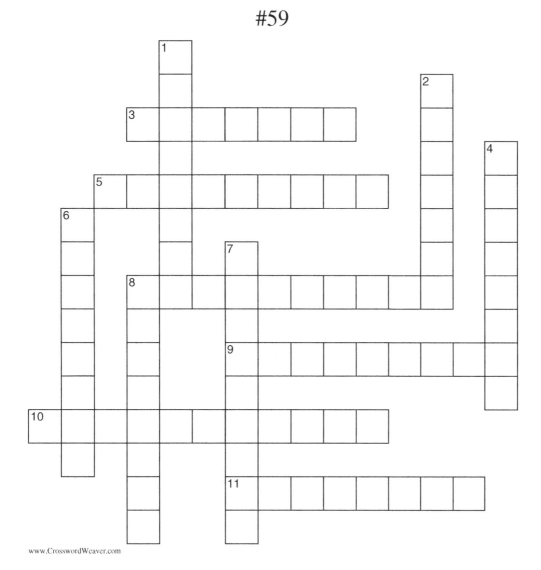

ACROSS

3 labor, parturition
5 of, relating to, or affecting the coccyx
8 to cut off the head of
9 of, relating to, or involving a nerve root
10 producing swelling
11 of or relating to diet

DOWN

1 abnormally swollen or dilated
2 weariness or exhaustion from labor, exertion, or stress
4 eyelid
6 a medical insignia bearing a representation of a staff with two entwined snakes and two wings at the top
7 murder of a father by his son or daughter
8 an increased excretion of urine

#60

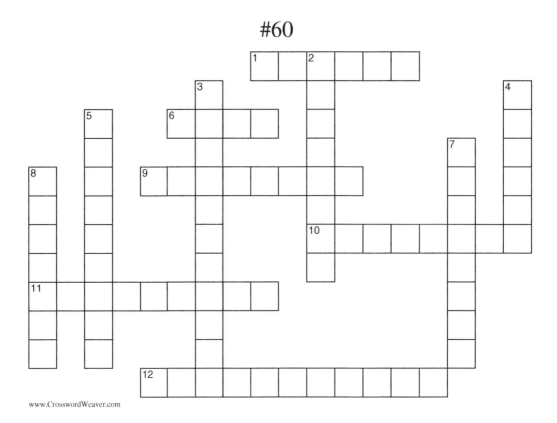

www.CrosswordWeaver.com

ACROSS

1 the protein shell of a virus particle that surrounds its nucleic acid

6 to undergo or cause (blood) to undergo a physiological change in which the hemoglobin becomes dissolved in the plasma

9 a phosphoprotein in egg yolk

10 a surgical instrument for cutting out circular sections (as of bone or corneal tissue)

11 a gonad containing both ovarian and testicular tissue

12 exerting or characterized by a direct influence on the secretory activity of the thyroid gland

DOWN

2 to diffuse through or penetrate something

3 surgical removal of all or part of the stomach

4 introduction of material into the stomach by a tube

5 surgical excision of selected portions of the frontal cortex of the brain esp. for relief of medically intractable epilepsy

7 the quality or state of being weak, feeble, or infirm; esp: physical weakness

8 likely to cause injury

#61

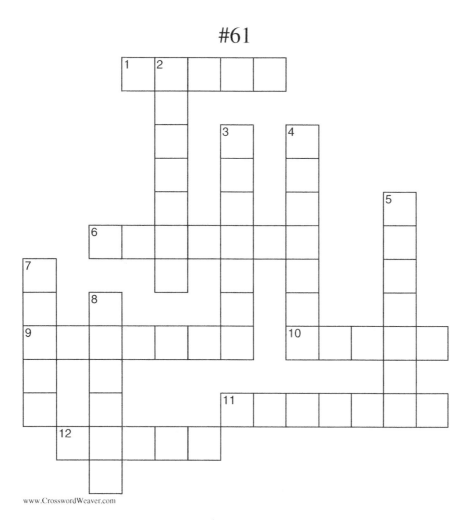

ACROSS

1 an ignorant or dishonest practitioner of medicine
6 of or relating to the diaphragm
9 the absense or impairment of the sense of taste
10 the blind pouch at the beginning of the large intestine into which the ilium opens from one side and which is continuous with the colon
11 curved like a bow
12 the largely cartilaginous projecting portion of the external ear

DOWN

2 a woman who has borne one child
3 a small tube for insertion into a body cavity, duct, or vessel
4 a person apparently sensitive to nonphysical forces
5 to divide (as a solution) into equal parts
7 a divice designed to encircle a tooth to hold a denture in place
8 a thick scar resulting from excessive growth of fibrous tissue and occurring esp. after burns or radiation injury

#62

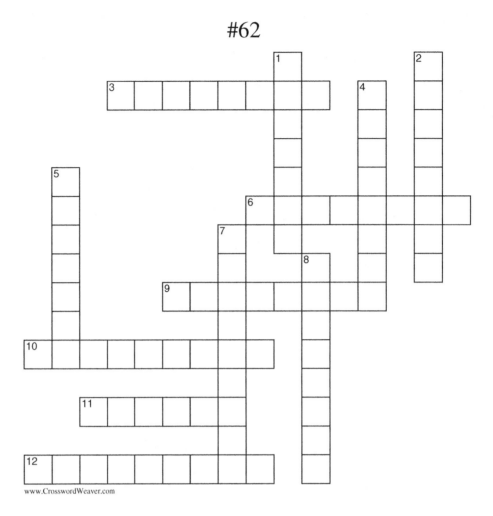

www.CrosswordWeaver.com

ACROSS

3 of, relating to, characterized by, or causing stenosis

6 a small slender straight or curved surgical knife with a sharp or blunt point

9 a mal-formed double fetus joined at the thorax and skull and having two equal faces looking in opposite directions

10 the intimate living together of two dissimilar organisms in a mutually beneficial relationship

11 a trembling or shaking usu. from physical weakness, emotional stress, or disease

12 lumpectomy

DOWN

1 the presence of an excess of fats or lipids in the blood

2 resembling the sound made by blowing across the mouth of an empty bottle

4 any disorder of pregnancy; esp. toxemia of pregnancy

5 a resonant sound heard in percussion (as of the abdomen)

7 a unit of mass and weight equal to 1/100 gram

8 a disease marked by dermatitis, gastrointestinal disorders, mental loss and associated with a diet deficient in niacin and protein

#63

ACROSS

1 having an adhesive quality
3 abnormal dryness of a body part or tissue (as the skin)
5 a chamber of the heart which receives blood from a corresponding atrium and from which blood is forced into the arteries
7 reduction of a medicinal solution to a fine spray
8 a region or area set off as distant
9 the state or fact of having borne offspring
10 relating to, involving, affecting or located in the region of the kidneys

DOWN

1 a substance in the gaseous state as distinguished from the liquid or solid state
2 a lame or partly disabled individual
4 a small hammer with a rubber head used in medical percussion
5 a small cavity or space in the tissues of an organism containing air or fluid
6 a small rigid jerky movement of the eye esp. as it jumps from fixation on one point to another (as in reading)

#64

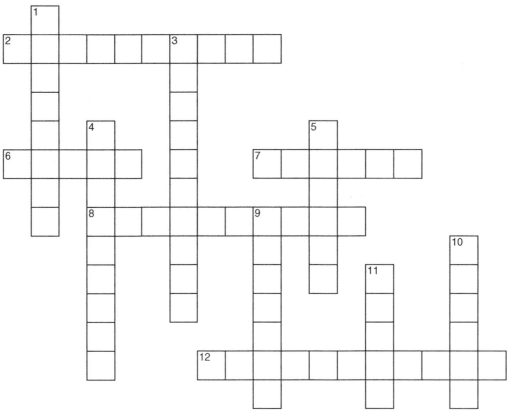

www.CrosswordWeaver.com

ACROSS

2 a process for copying graphic matter by the action of light on an electrically charged surface in which the latent image is developed with a resinous powder

6 a chronic problem patient who does not respond to treatment (usu. disparaging)

7 an inability to coordinate voluntary muscular movements that is symptomatic of some nervous disorders

8 the settling of blood in relatively lower parts of an organ or the body due to impaired or absent circulation

12 parrot fever

DOWN

1 any of various synthetic or naturally occurring analogs of vitamin A

3 abnormal deficiency or absence of sweating

4 pain in the head--called also headache

5 a thin plate or layer esp. of an anatomical part

9 the white of an egg

10 inability to walk caused by a defect in muscular coordination

11 an enveloping case or sheath of an anatomical part

#65

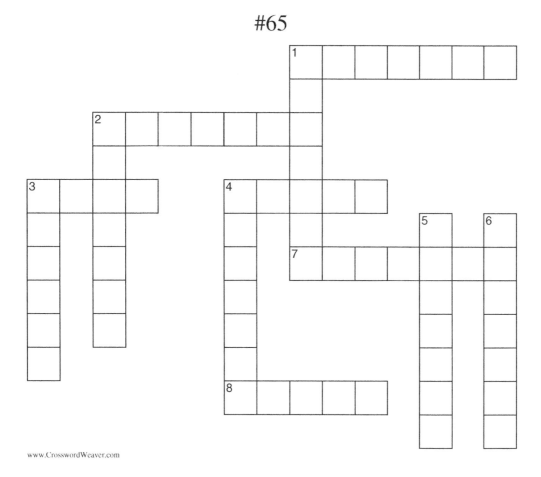

ACROSS

1 a white or yellow hard brittle wax
2 a dead body ; spec: one intended for dissection
3 heel
4 a tubular anatomical passage or channel: duct
7 an individual, organ, or part consisting of tissues of diverse genetic constitution
8 the upper part of the human cranium

DOWN

1 marked by long duration, by frequent recurrence over a long time, and often by slowly progressing seriousness : not acute
2 a thickening of or a hard thickened area on the skin
3 of or relating to the abdominal cavity
4 of or relating to heat
5 earwax
6 sedative

#66

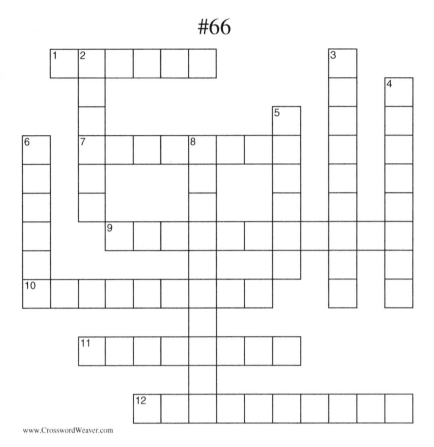

www.CrosswordWeaver.com

ACROSS

1 to reduce the intensity or sensitivity of: make dull

7 a disease of the eye marked by increased pressure within the eyeball that can result in damage to the optic disk and gradual loss of vision

9 a green pigment that occurs in bile and is formed by breakdown of hemoglobin

10 dread of or aversion to novelty

11 central nervous system

12 existing at or dating from birth

DOWN

2 the point of junction of the coronal and sagittal sutures of the skull

3 not sufficiently developed to survive outside the uterus

4 characterized by essentially identical genes

5 to hold (as liquid) in the mouth or throat and agitate with air from the lungs

6 a gluey protein substance esp. of wheat flour that causes dough to be sticky

8 an inflammatory swelling or sore caused by exposure (as of the feet or hands) to cold

#67

www.CrosswordWeaver.com

ACROSS

3 dislocation of an anatomical part
4 an irresistable impulse to start fires
7 hernistion of the rectum through a defect in the intervening fascia into the vagina
8 the study of the general principles of scientific classification
9 a small muscle on each side of the nose that constricts the nasal aperture
10 facilitating the urinary excretion of salt and esp.of sodium ion
11 notched or toothed on the edge

DOWN

1 abnormal dryness of a body part or tissue (as the skin)
2 to make involuntary stops and repititions in speaking
5 a condition characterized by abnormally small and imperfectly developed extremities
6 containing, consisting of, or being pus

#68

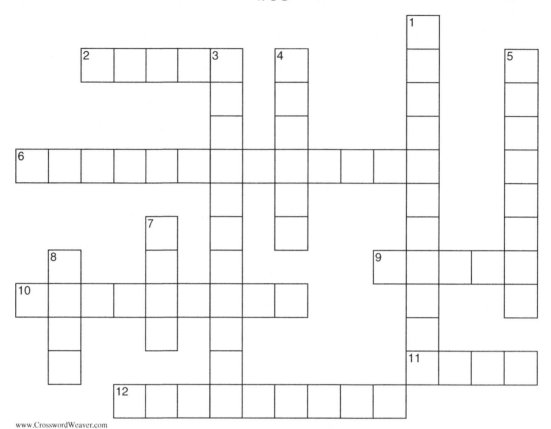

www.CrosswordWeaver.com

ACROSS

2 the property of a thing that affects the olfactory organs: odor

6 having a yellowish discoloration

9 to respond to a stimulus

10 inhibiting uterine contractions

11 hip joint, hip

12 dysfunction of the sense of taste

DOWN

1 of, relating to or being epileptic seizures precipitated by music

3 characterized by piercing or stabbing sensations

4 any of various solid steroid alcohols (as cholesterol) widely distributed in animal and plant lipids

5 to engage in sexual intercourse

7 castrate : also : spay

8 a state of profound unconsciousness caused by distress, injury, or poison

#69

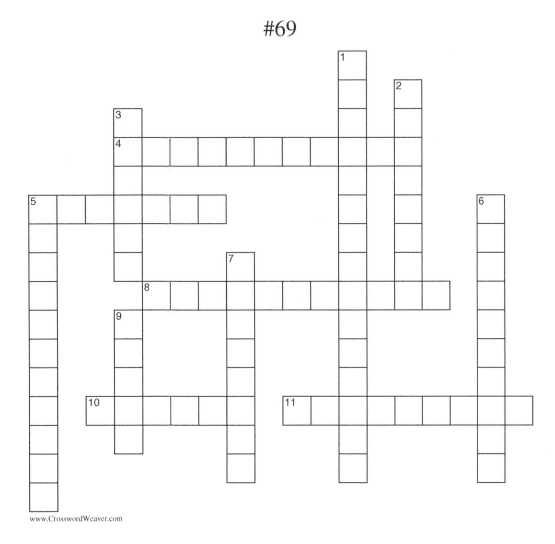

www.CrosswordWeaver.com

ACROSS

4 the surgical formation of an opening between a renal pelvis and the outside of the body
5 to exclude from consciousness
8 occurring about or surrounding the crown of a tooth
10 to return or restore to consciousness or life
11 of , relating to, being, or lying in the region of the inferior part of the sphenoid bone

DOWN

1 mental processes outside the main stream of consciousness but sometimes available to it
2 the presence of glucose in the blood
3 a cavity within a bone (as the maxilla) or hollow organ (as the stomach)
5 characterized by, allowing, or being a backward flow (as of blood)
6 a gastric calculus
7 a space between teeth in a jaw
9 an official or standard collection of drug formulas and descriptions

#70

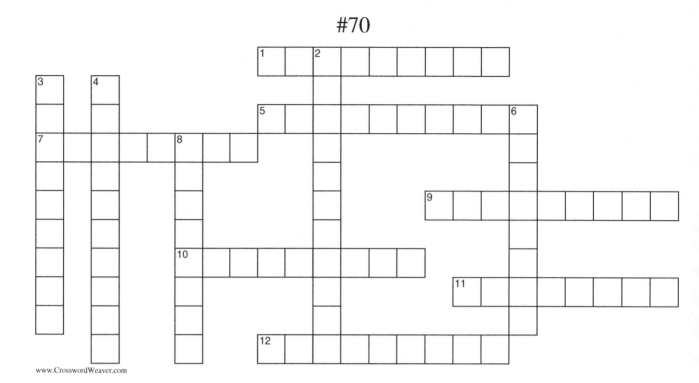

www.CrosswordWeaver.com

ACROSS

1 a condition of having fetid breath
5 incapable of being felt by touch
7 to draw by suction
9 surgical removal of a lobe of an organ (as a lung) or gland (as the thyroid) specif: excision of a lobe of the lung
10 to cripple by cutting the leg tendons
11 a dark greenish mass of desqamated cells, mucus, and bile that accumulates in the bowel of a fetus and is typically discharged shortly after birth
12 derived from two ova: dizygotic

DOWN

2 a lipoma containing fibrous tissue
3 a specialist in anatomy
4 a condition of arrested development in which an organ or part remains below the normal size or in an immature state
6 a science that deals with the improvement (as by control of human mating) of hereditary qualities of a race or breed
8 being without functioning kidneys

#71

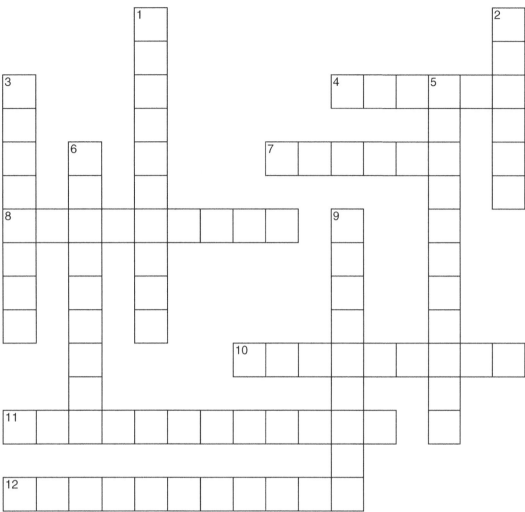

www.CrosswordWeaver.com

ACROSS

4 a tumor arising from glial cells
7 a spasmodic variation in the size of the pupil of the eye caused by a tremor of the iris
8 hemiplegia plus paralysis of a limb on the opposite side
10 lying or occurring anterior to the tibia
11 containing both mucus and pus
12 sleep of excessive depth or duration

DOWN

1 to take in and utilize as nourishment : absorb into the system
2 exhibiting opacity : not allowing passage of radiant energy
3 the action or result of binding or tying
5 severe and intractable constipation
6 not accompanied or characterized by jaundice
9 abnormally low pressure of the intraocular fluid

#72

ACROSS

1 a small muscle on each side of the nose that constricts the nasal aperture

7 excision of the cardiac portion of the stomach

8 a colorless odorless inert gaseous element

9 an inflammatory swelling or sore

10 tending to soothe or soften

11 a stricture or narrowing esp. of a canal or vessel (as the aorta)

DOWN

2 acute or chronic pain caused by muscle strain in lower back

3 upper portion of a bodily part

4 a large vesicle or blister

5 the fourth letter of the Greek alphabet

6 a convoluted ridge between anatomical grooves

9 any of generally abnormal sounds heard on auscultation

#73

www.CrosswordWeaver.com

ACROSS

3 abnormally high blood pressure
5 discharge of blood secretions , and tissue debris from the uterus at monthly intervals
7 resembling or functioning as a valve
10 inflammation of synovial membrane
11 digestive tract
12 having an affinity for lymphocytes

DOWN

1 thick fluid composed of exudate containing white blood cells
2 relating to the tarsus
4 abnormal slowness of thought or action
6 to stop in the early stages
8 cell that engulfs and consumes foreign material
9 closed sac with distinct membrane and develops abnormally in body cavity or structure

#74

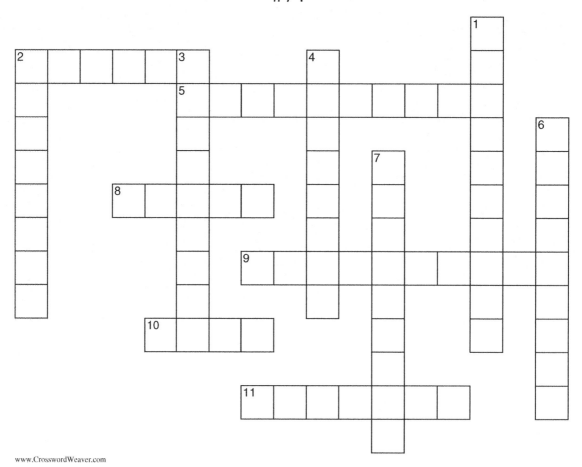

www.CrosswordWeaver.com

ACROSS

2 exhibiting or capable of movement

5 a mixed tumor containing both fibrous and muscle tissue

8 belch

9 one of five children or offspring born at one birth

10 a canopy or enclosure placed over the head and shoulders to retain vapors or oxygen during medical administration

11 a heavy-duty forceps for removing small pieces of bone or tough tissue

DOWN

1 one of four offspring born at one birth

2 being in the state of dying: approaching death

3 a light stroking movement used in massage

4 exaggerated forward curvature of the lumbar and cervical regions of the spinal column

6 of or relating to the muscular coat of the intestinal wall

7 one of seven offspring born at one birth

#75

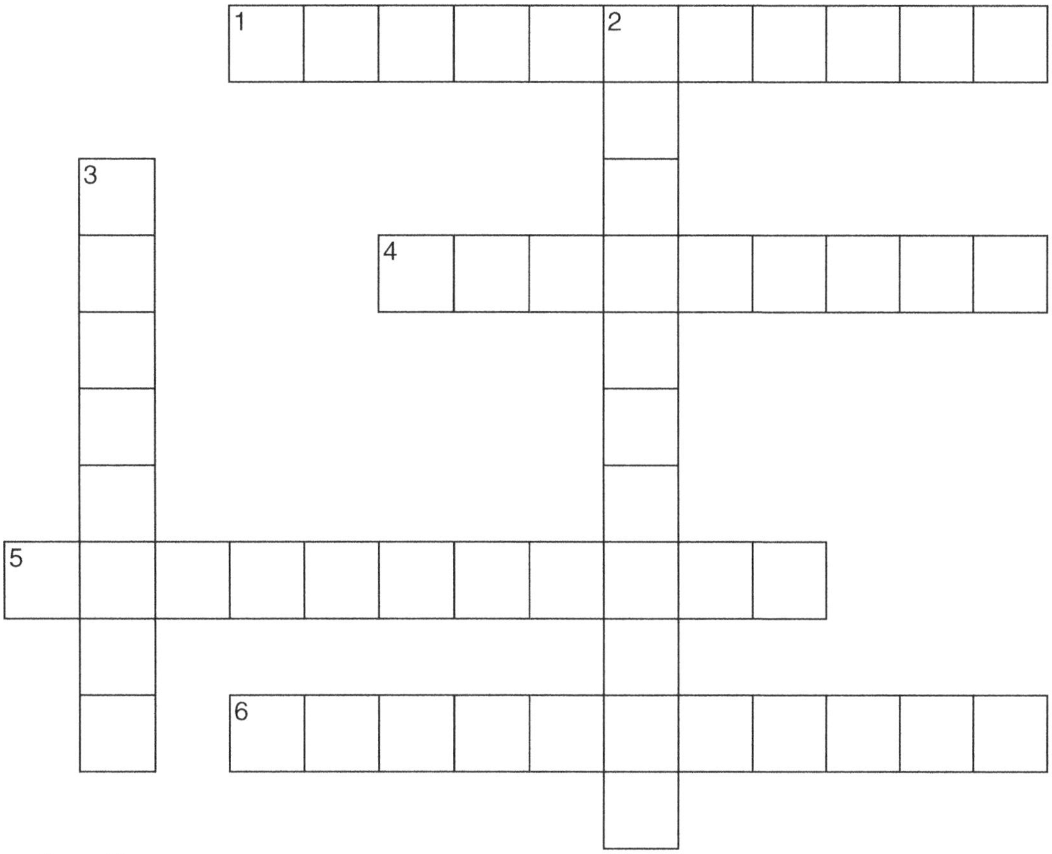

ACROSS

1 situated or extending between the ribs

4 sexual excitement associated with urine or with urination

5 the description or study of the phenomena of death and of psychological mechanisms for coping with them

6 the apparent production of motion in objects (as by a spiritualistic medium) without contact or other physical means

DOWN

2 a green pigment that occurs in bile and is formed by breakdown of hemoglobin

3 a discharge of pus

www.CrosswordWeaver.com

Solution:

#1

```
            E       M E A T U S
            G       U
    E C T O P I C   C     T   P
            A       O X I D E   S
            R       I     C     S
    O       T       D           T
    V       R                   I
    O V A R I A N               F
    I       T           V       E
    D   E C Z E M A     A       R
                        S       O
                                U
                                S
```

Solution:

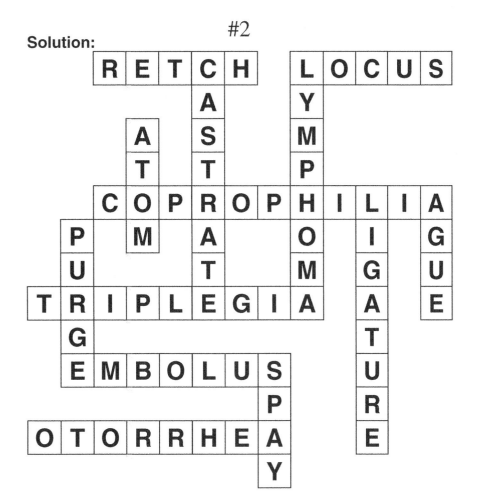

Solution:

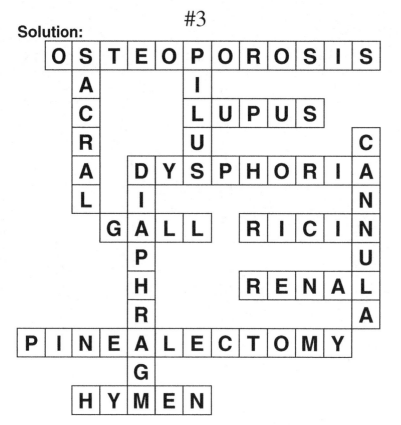

O S T E O P O R O S I S

S A C R A L

P I L U S

L U P U S

C A N N U L A

D Y S P H O R I A

D I A P H R A G M

G A L L

R I C I N

R E N A L

P I N E A L E C T O M Y

H Y M E N

Solution:

#4

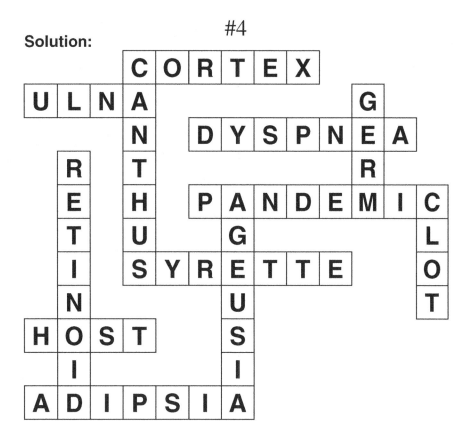

Solution:

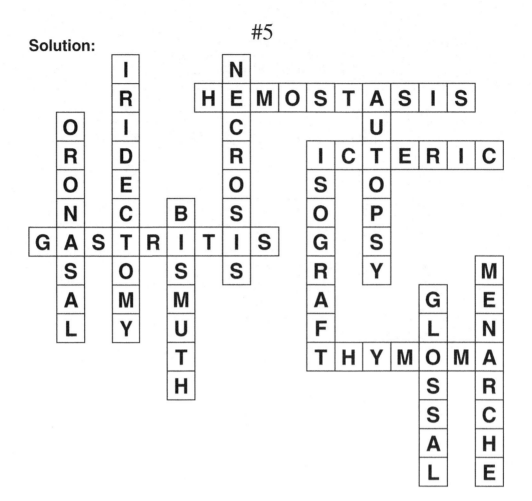

Solution:

#6

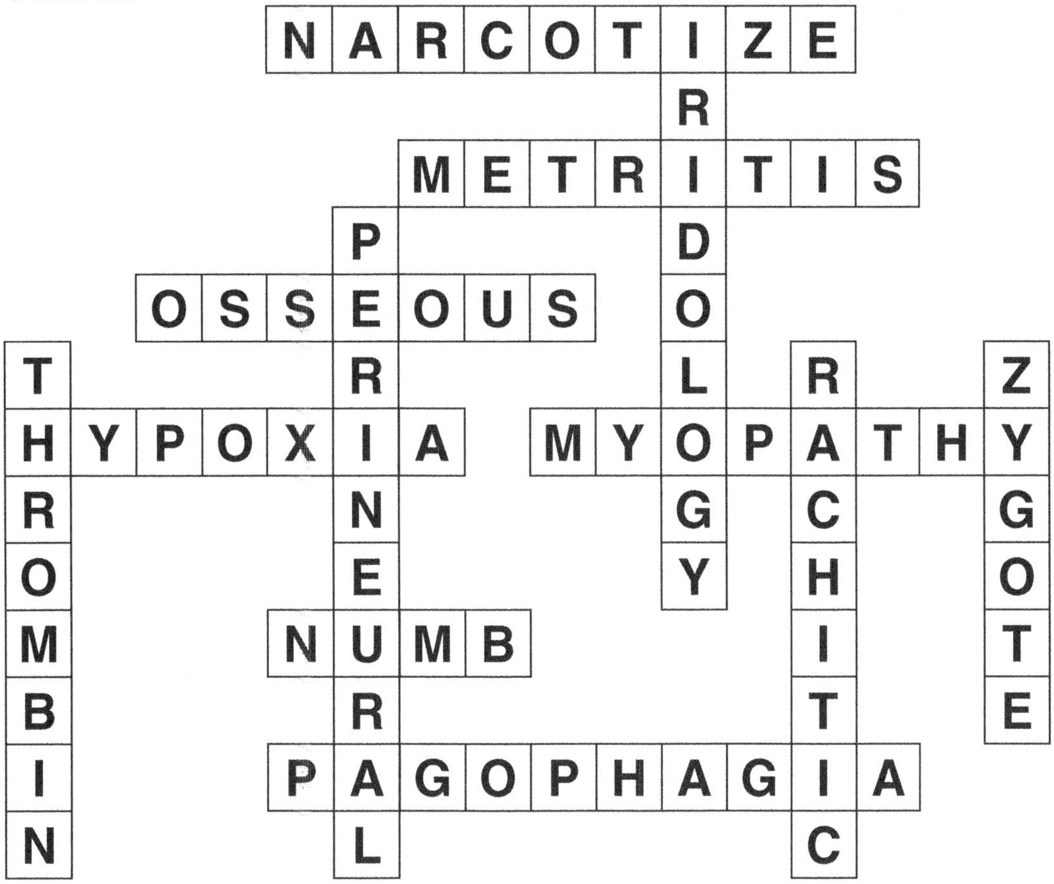

NARCOTIZE

METRITIS

OSSEOUS

HYPOXIA MYOPATHY

NUMB

PAGOPHAGIA

Down words (crossing):
- IRIDOLOGY
- THROMBIN
- PERINEURAL
- ZYGOTE
- RACHITIC

Solution:

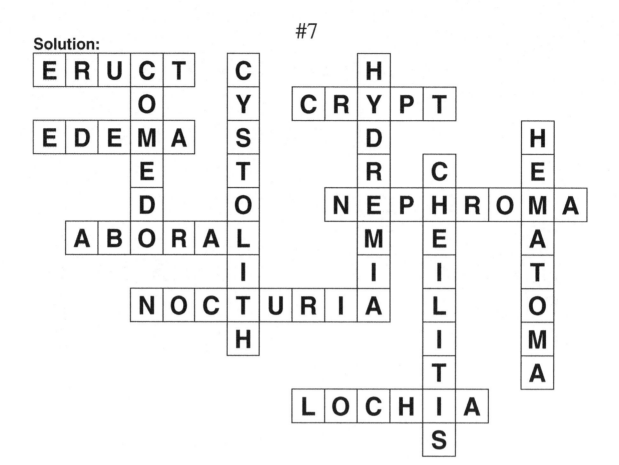

Solution:

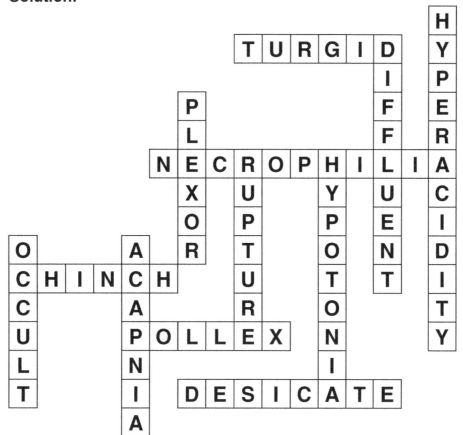

Solution:

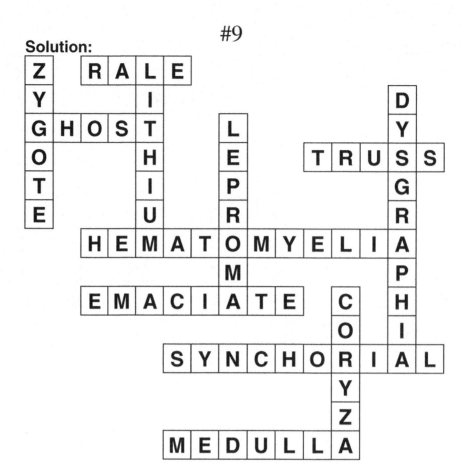

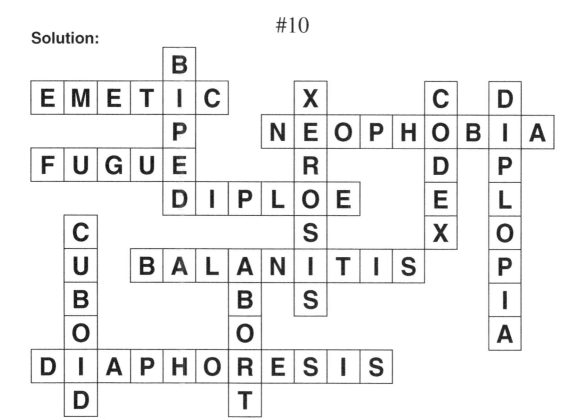

Solution:

#11

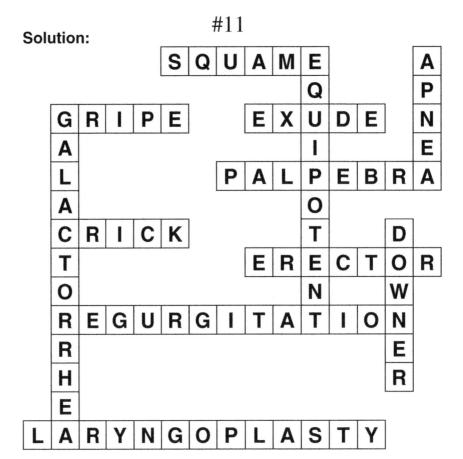

Solution:

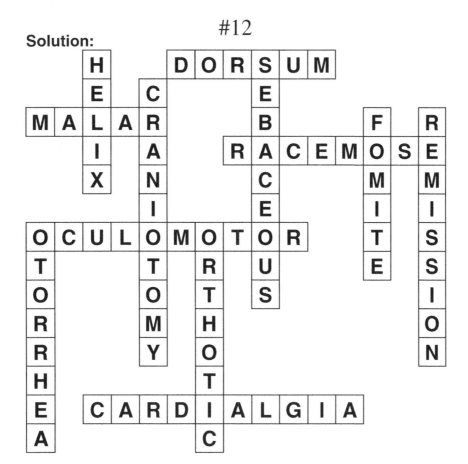

Solution:

#13

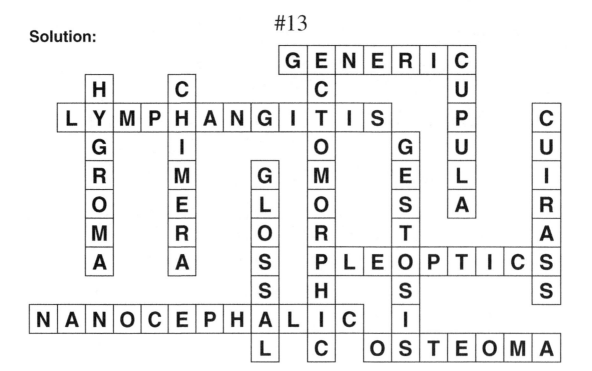

Solution:

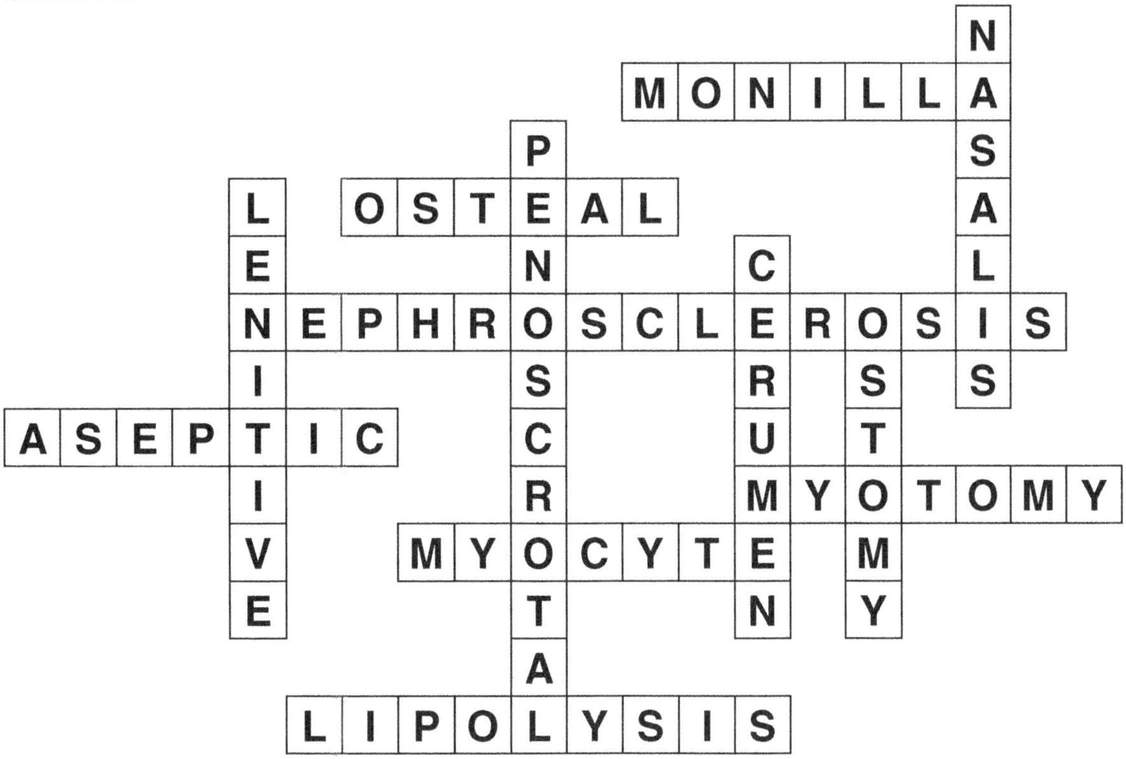

#14

MONILLA NASALIS

OSTEAL

LENITIVE

NEPHROSCLEROSIS

ASEPTIC

PENOSCROTAL

CERUMEN

MYOTOMY

CYSTOMY

MYOCYTE

LIPOLYSIS

Solution:

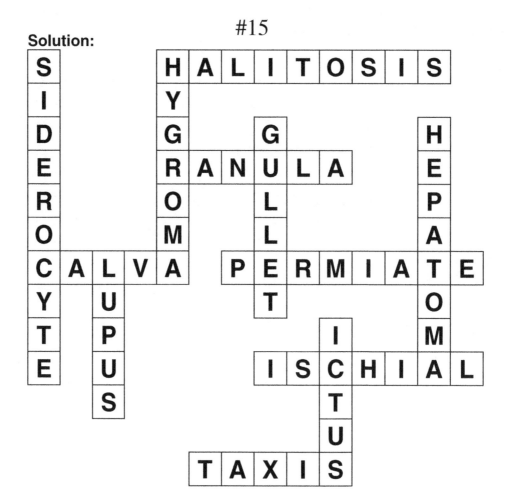

Solution:

```
H E T E R O T O P I C
        H               C           M
      B I O T I C       H           A
    R   Z               L           C
Z O O N O S I S         O X Y N T I C
    U   M               R           R
    L   M           U M B R O       O
O L I G E M I A         S   U       C
    E   T               I   B       Y
    A   I               S   O       T
    U   O C C I P U T   S           E
```

Solution:

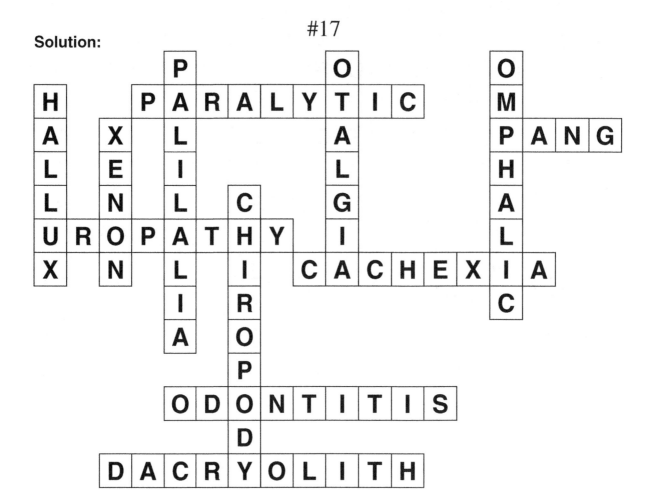

Solution:

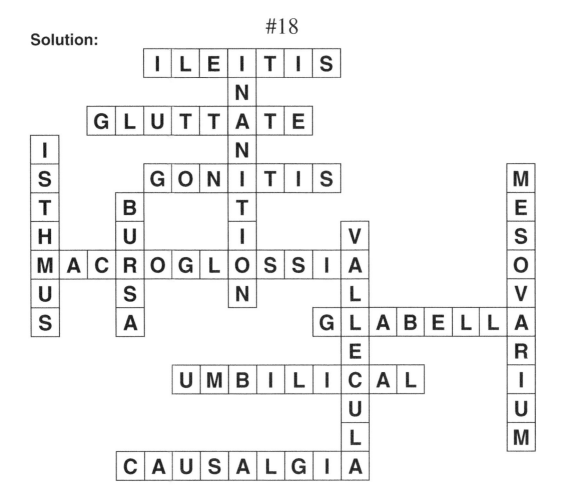

#19

Solution:

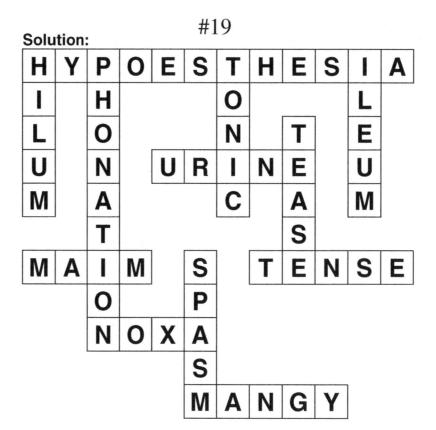

Solution:

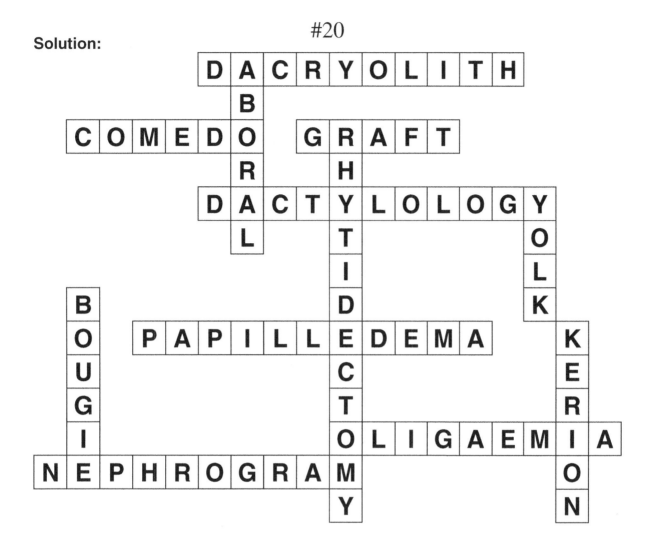

#21

Solution:

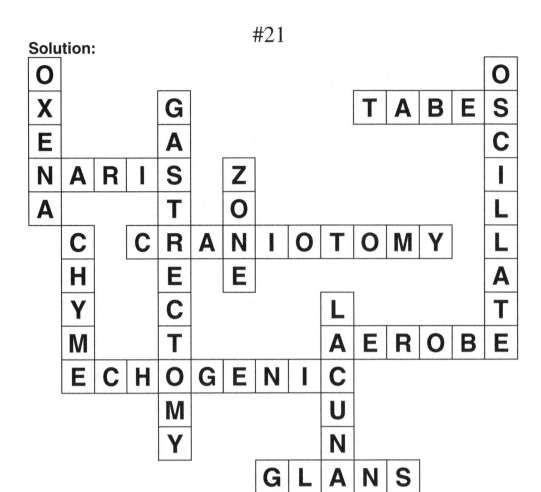

Solution:

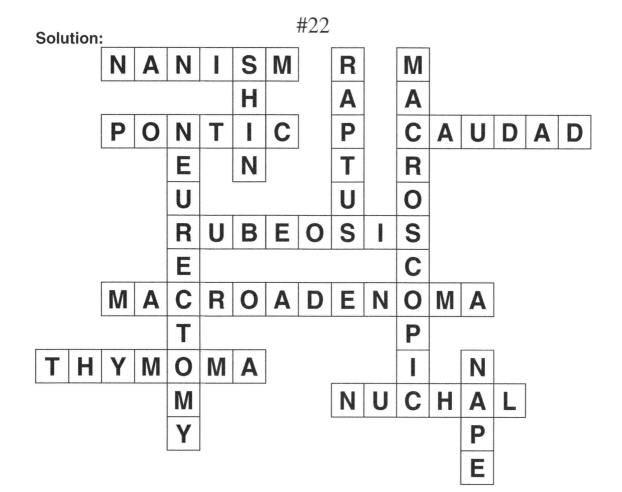

Solution:

#23

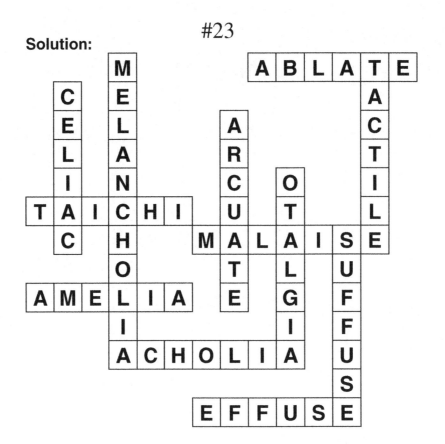

#24

Solution:

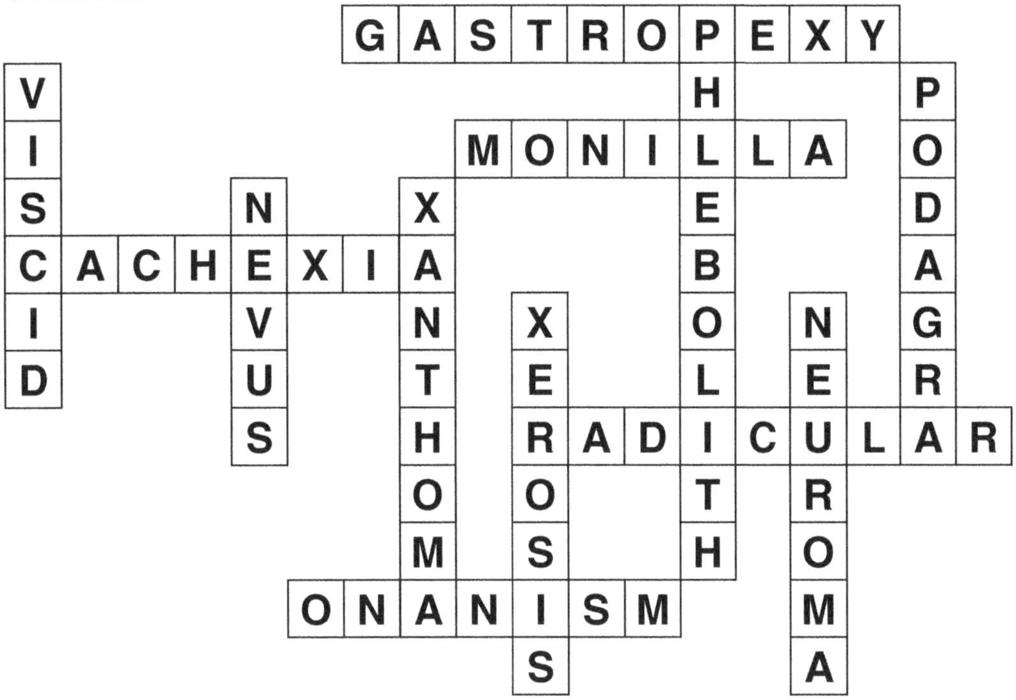
GASTROPEXY
VISCID
PHLEBOLITH
PODAGRA
MONILLA
NEVUS
XANTHOMA
CACHEXIA
XEROSIS
NEUROMA
RADICULAR
ONANISM

Solution:

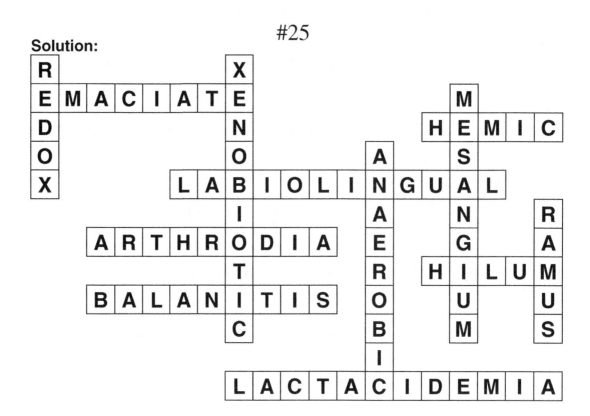

Solution:

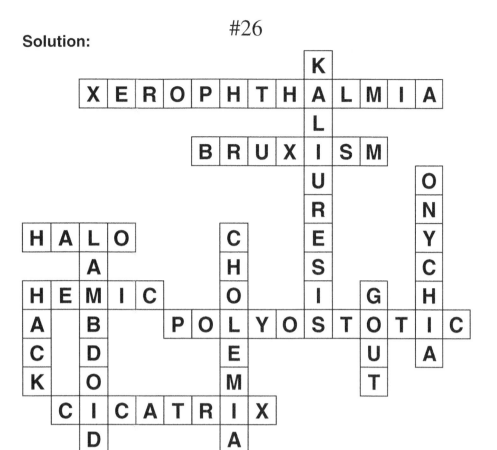

Solution:

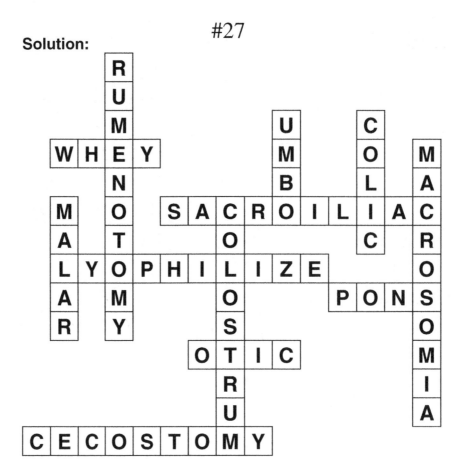

Solution:

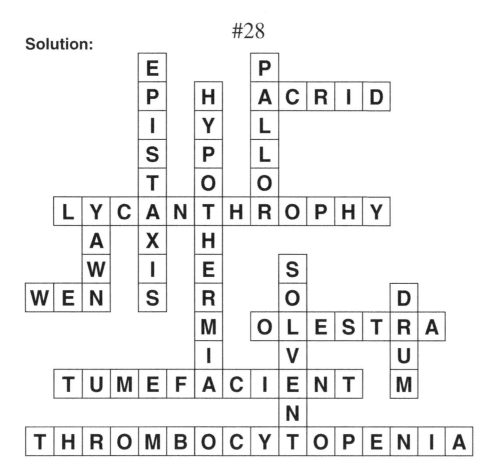

Solution:

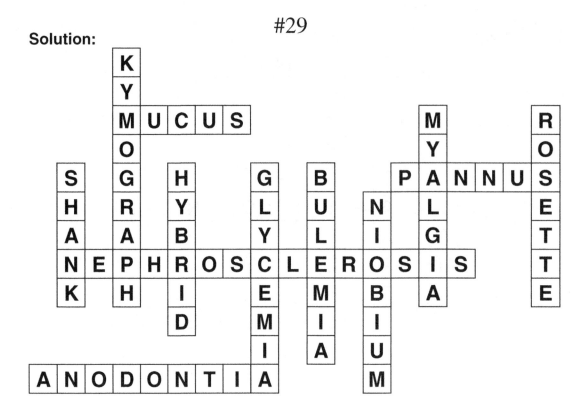

Solution:

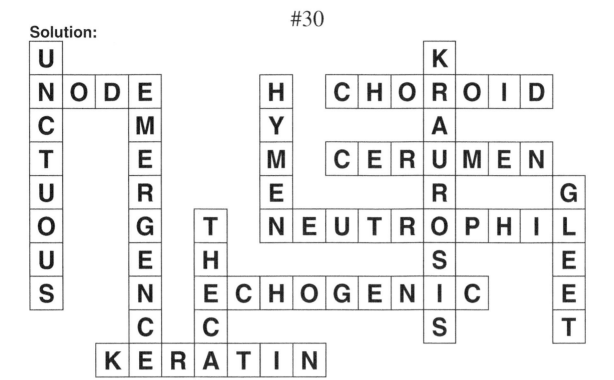

Solution:

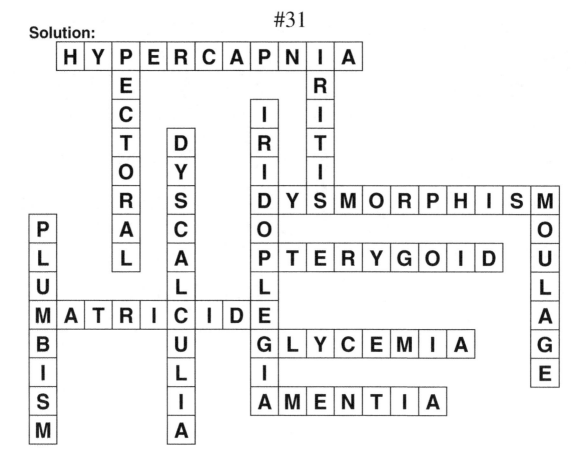

Solution:

```
                R
      P E S C A R V U S             V
              T   R           Y     E
              R   Y     T E N O D E S I S
  C           U   P     R   D       I     A
  Y           S   T     A   A       C     L
  C           I   I     N   C       A     I
  L           O   T     S   T       N     C
  O X Y N T   I C       G   Y   E C T H Y M A
  P           S         E   L       L
  S                     N           I
                        E           S
                                    M
```

Across / Down entries:
- PES CARVUS
- RETRUSION
- CRYPTITIS
- TENODESIS
- TRANSGENE
- TEDACTYL
- VESICAN
- SALICYLISM
- OXYNTIC
- CYCLOPS
- ECTHYMA
- PORCINE

Solution:

#33

```
                    I                   L
           O        N          O        A        I
           D        C          X        C        M
           N        R          Y        R        P
           T        U    T A M P O N A D E
           A        S         T        A        E
   H Y A L I T I S          C        L        T
           G        A          I                 I
           I        T          C                 G
           A        I                            O
                    O
                    N
```

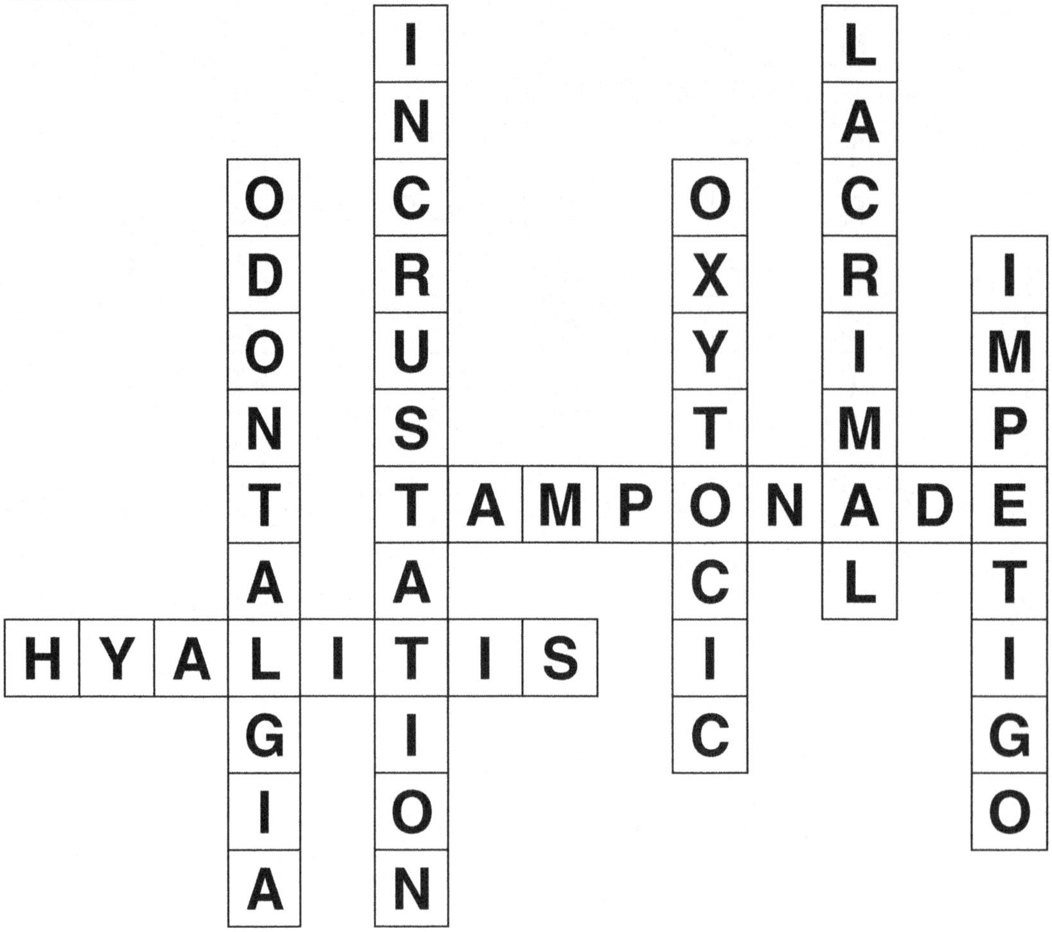

Solution:

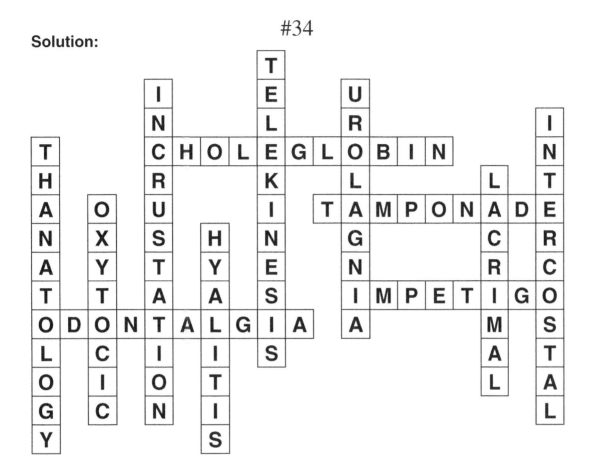

Solution:

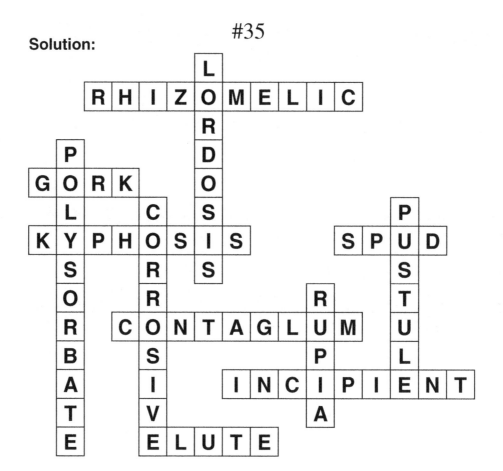

Solution:

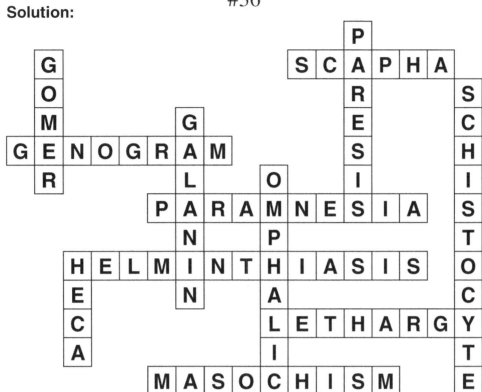

Solution:

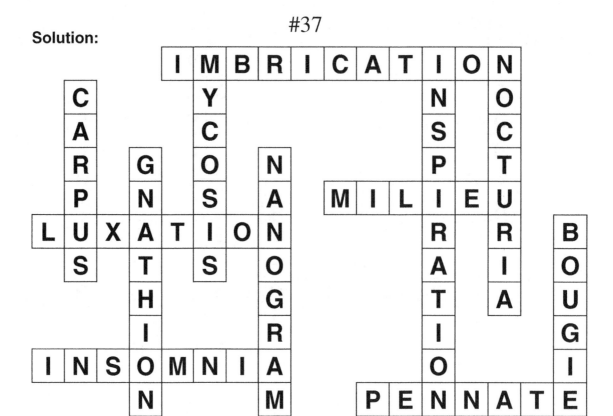

Solution:

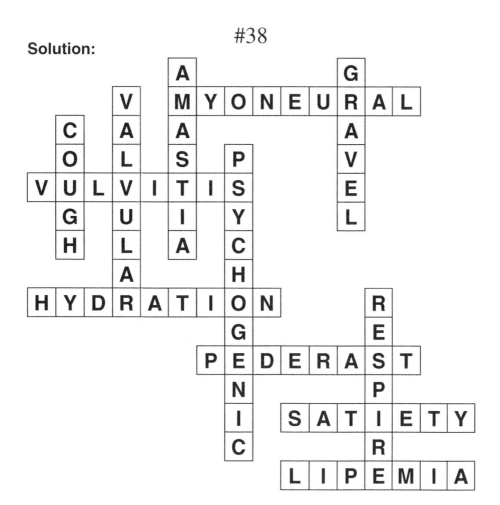

Solution:

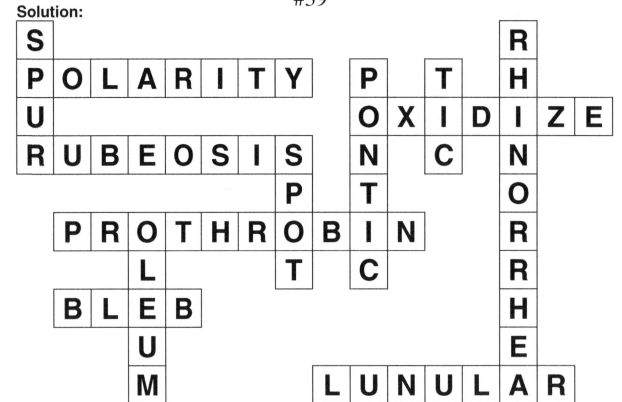

Solution:

```
                    S A P P H I S T
          D     E             A                   G
        F I B R O C Y T E     L                   L
          L     O             A                   O
          D     T             B   B L U E S       S
          O     I             R                   S
              O C C U L T     A                   O
                      U       S                   L
          C R Y O N I C S     I                   A
                      S       O                   L
            R E G U R G I T A N T                 I
                      V                           A
      H Y P O F E R R E M I A
```

Solution:

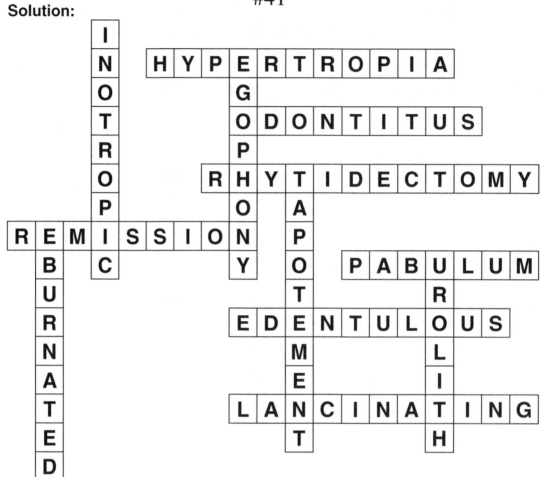

Solution:

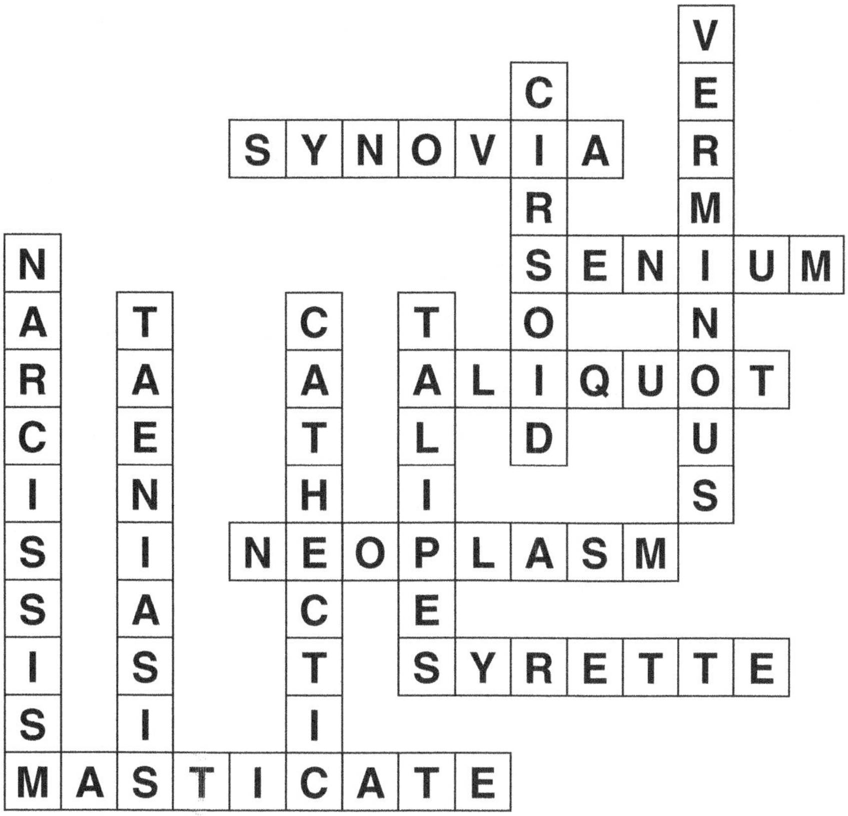

SYNOVIA

VERMINOUS

CIRSOID

SENIUM

NARCISSISSISM

TAENIASIS

CATHCTIT

TALIDE

ALIQUOT

NEOPLASM

SYRETTE

MASTICATE

Solution:

```
                              O S T E C T O M Y
                                  H
                      G   C Y S T O T O M Y
                      E         O
              L A B R U M       L
          L   I             H   E
          A   I N N E R V A T E L
          L   C         L       I
    S A L P I N G E C T O M Y   T   H
          T   R         Y       H   E
          I   I         O       I   M
          O   S   I C H T H Y O S I S
          N   S         P       A   P
                        H       S   T
                        I           Y
                        L           S
                        I           I
                        Z           S
                    T E N O D E S I S
```

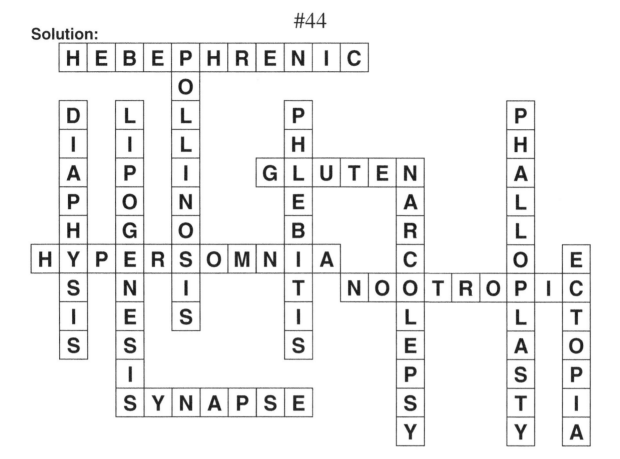

Solution:

Solution:

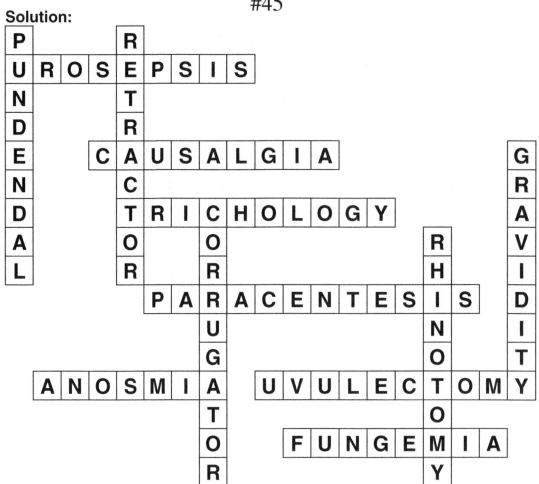

Solution:

#46

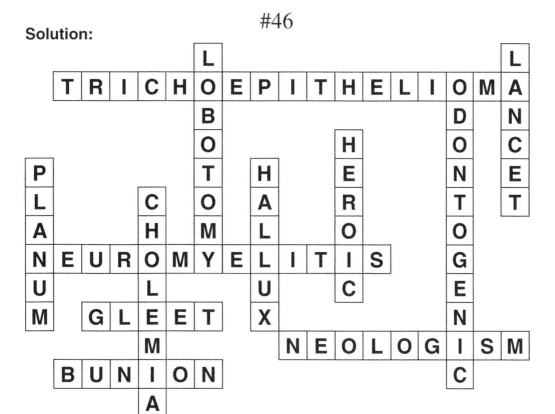

Solution:

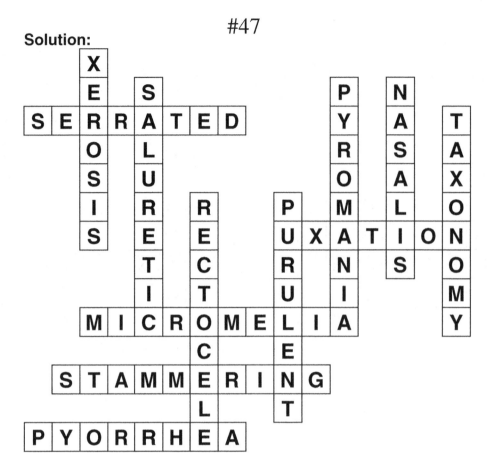

#48

Solution:

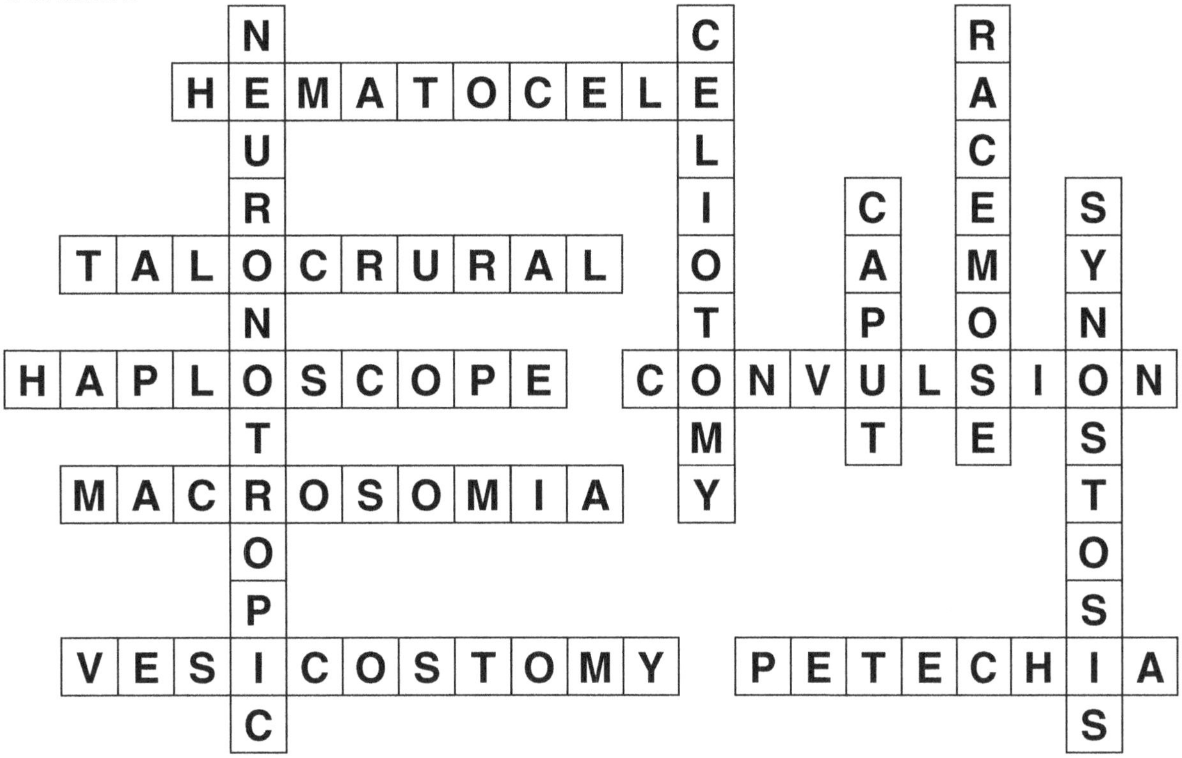

Across and down answers:

HEMATOCELE

TALOCRURAL

HAPLOSCOPE

CONVULSION

MACROSOMIA

VESICOSTOMY

PETECHIA

Down: NEURONOTROPIC, CELIOTOMY, CAPUT, RACEMOSE, SYNOSTOSIS

#49

Solution:

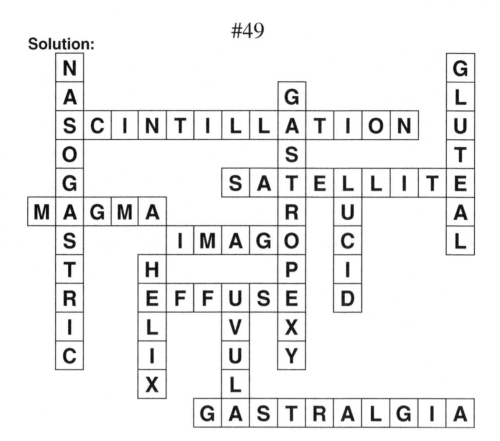

Solution:

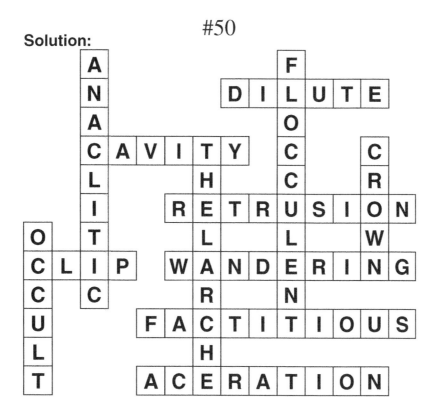

Solution:

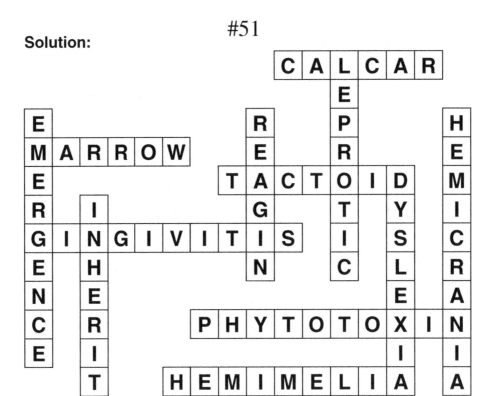

Solution:

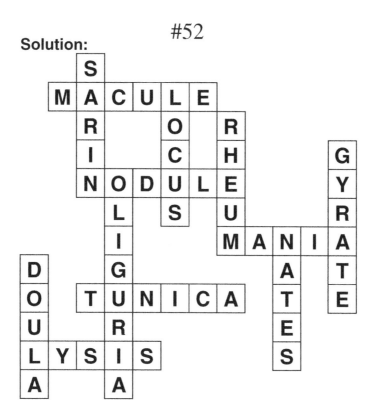

Solution:

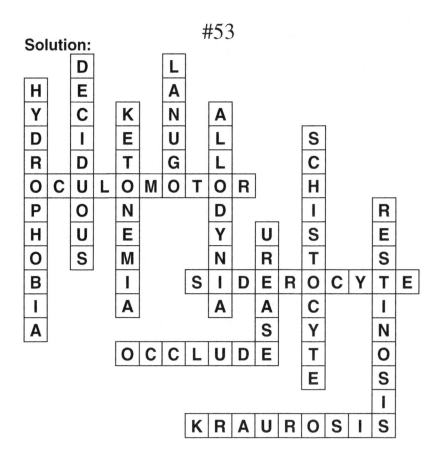

Solution:

#54

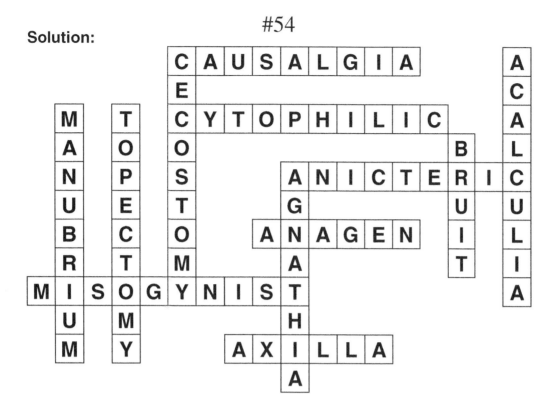

Solution:

#55

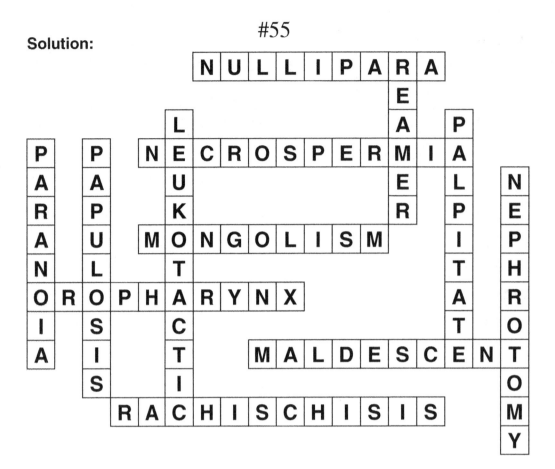

Solution:

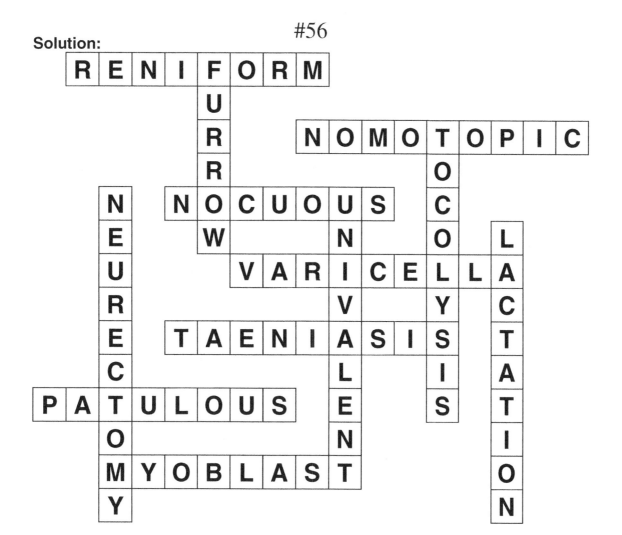

Solution:

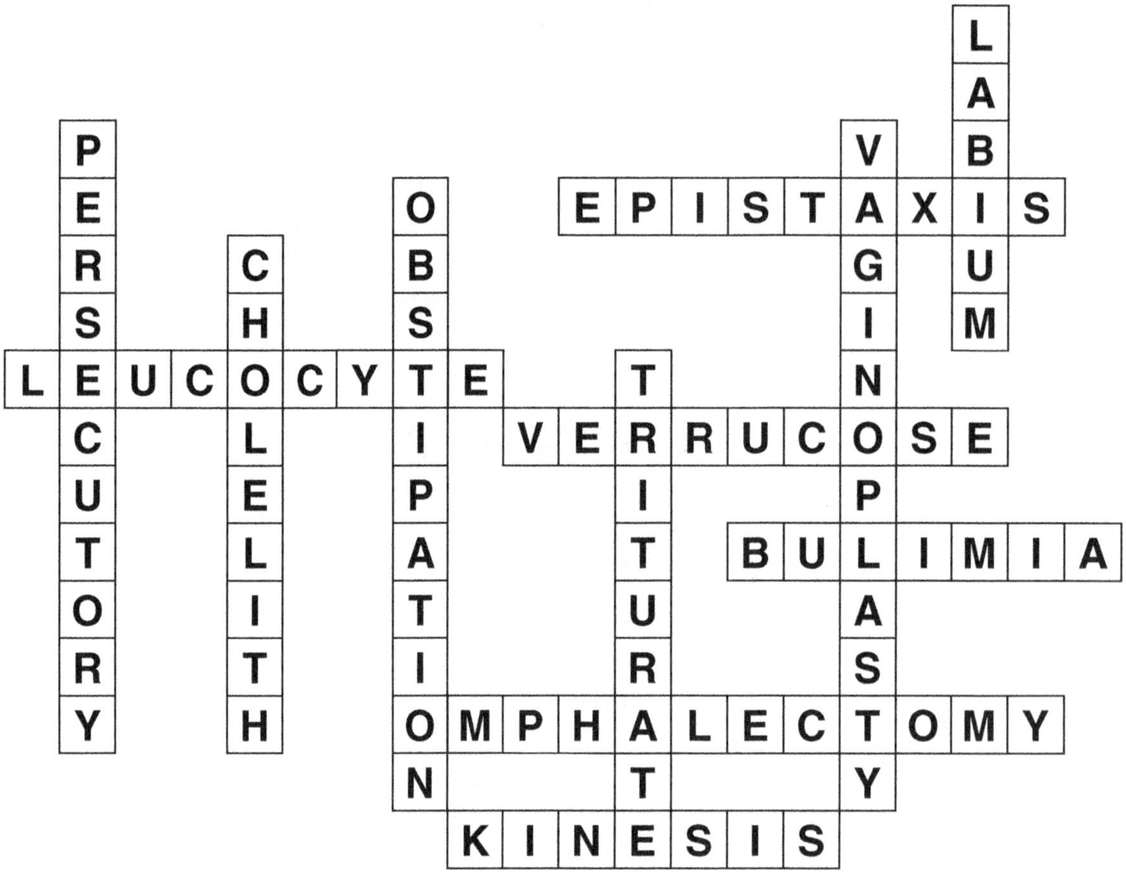

LABIUM

PERSECUTORY

LEUCOCYTE

CHOLELITH

OBSTIPATION

EPISTAXIS

VAGINOPLASTY

VERRUCOSE

TRITURATT

BULIMIA

OMPHALECTOMY

KINESIS

Solution:

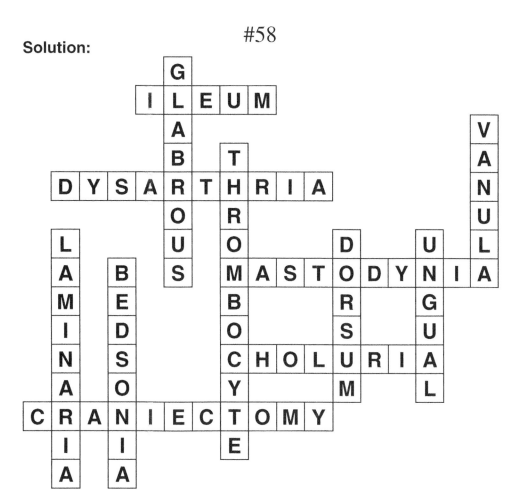

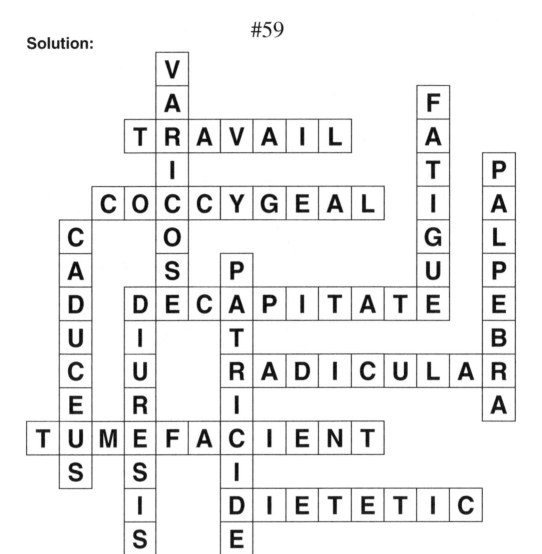

Solution:

Solution:

#60

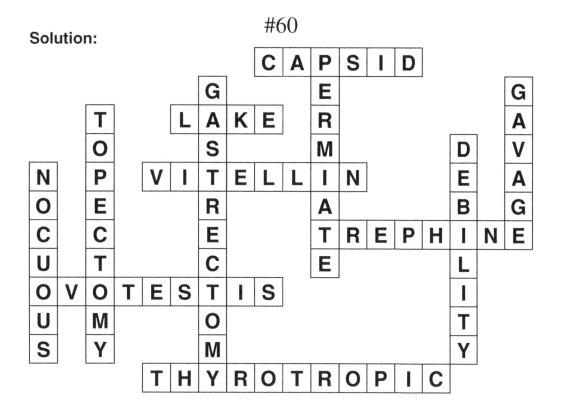

Solution:

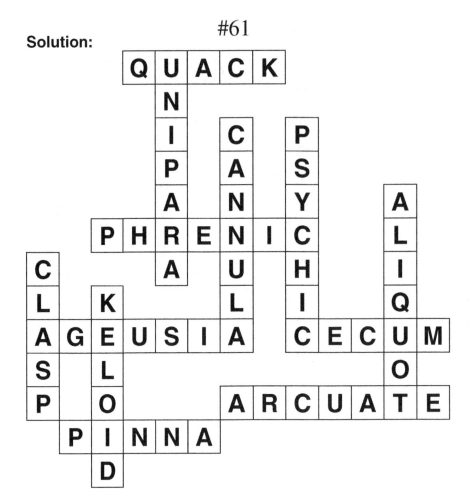

Solution:

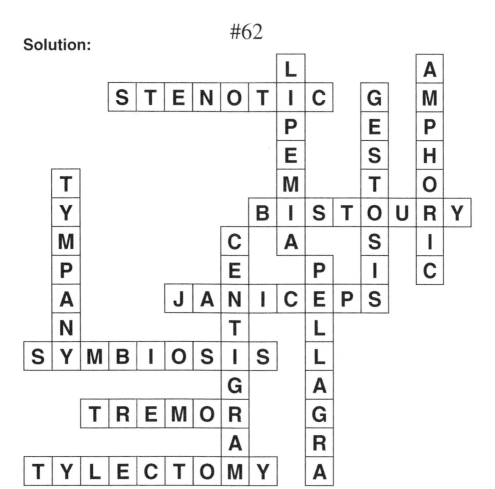

Solution:

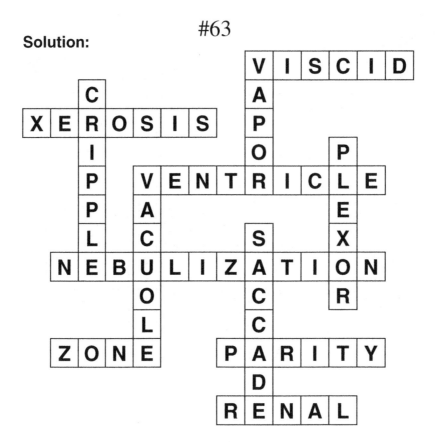

#64

Solution:

A crossword puzzle solution grid containing the following words:

- XEROGRAPHY
- RETINOID
- GOMER
- ATAXIA
- ANHYDROSIS
- CEPHALALGIA
- HYPOSTASIS
- LAMINA
- ALBUMIN
- PSITTACOSIS
- THECA
- ABASIA

Solution:

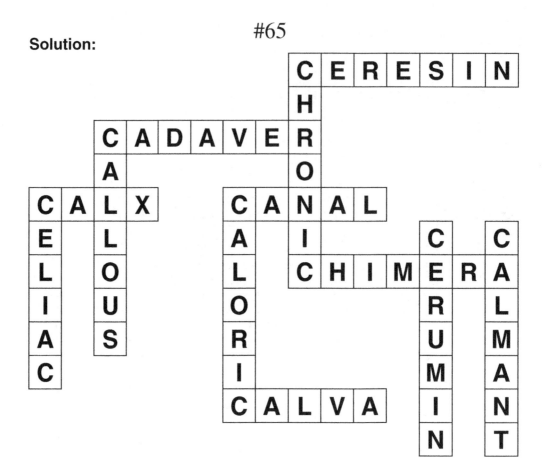

Solution: #66

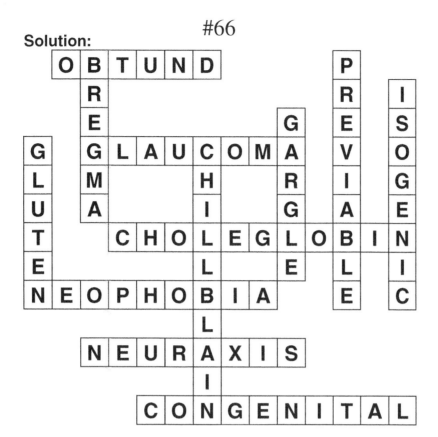

Solution:

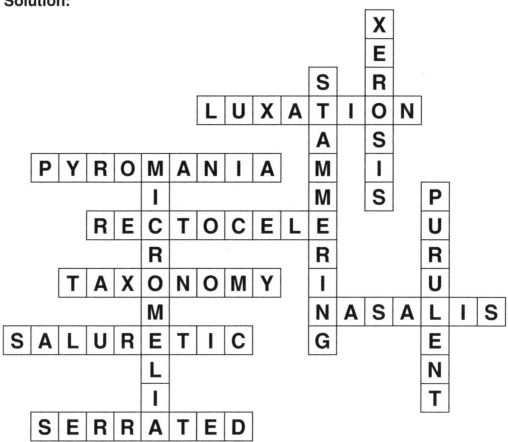

Solution:

```
          S M E L L     S         M           C
                  A     T         U           O
                  N     E         S           P
  X A N T H O C H R O M I C       I           U
                  I     R         C           L
              G   N     O         O           A
          C   E   A     L         G   R E A C T
  T O C O L Y T I C               E           E
          M   D   T               N
          A       I               I   C O X A
              D Y S G E U S I A
```

#69

Solution:

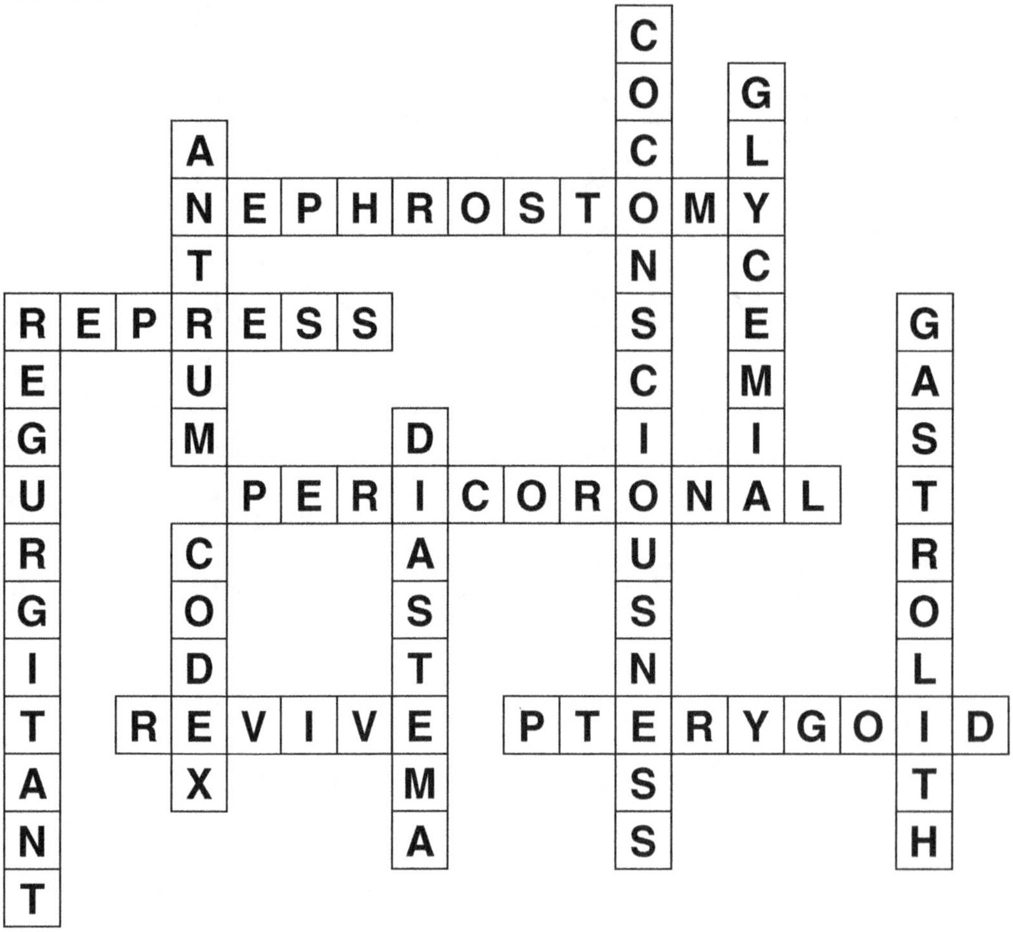

NEPHROSTOMY
REPRESS
PERICORONAL
REVIVE
PTERYGOID
CONSCIOUSNESS
GLYCEMIA
ANTRUM
REGURGITANT
DIASTEMA
CODEX
GASTROLITH

Solution:

#70

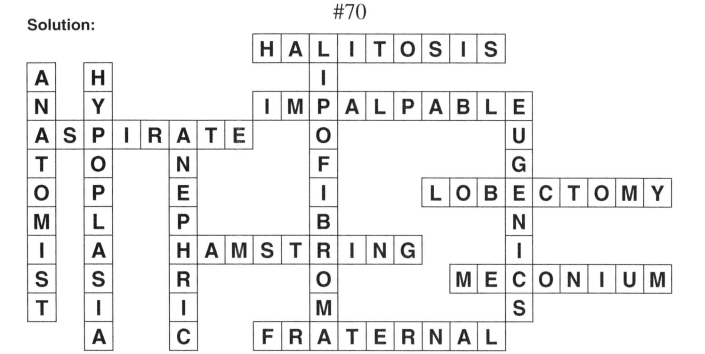

Solution:

ASSIMILATE (down, crossing)

GLIOMA

OPAQUE

LIGATURE

ANICTERIC

HIPPUS

OBSTIPATION

TRIPLEGIA

HYPOTONIA

PRETIBIAL

MUCOPURULENT

HYPERSOMNIA

Solution:

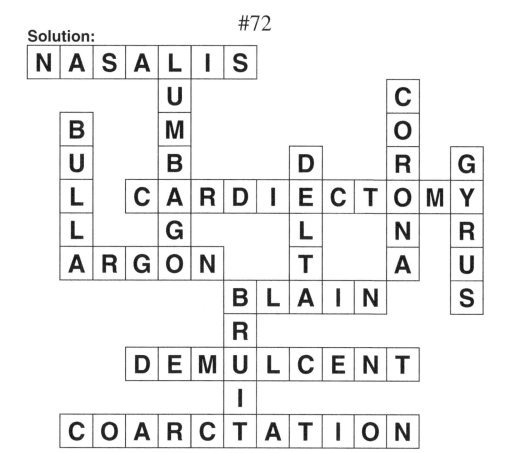

Solution:

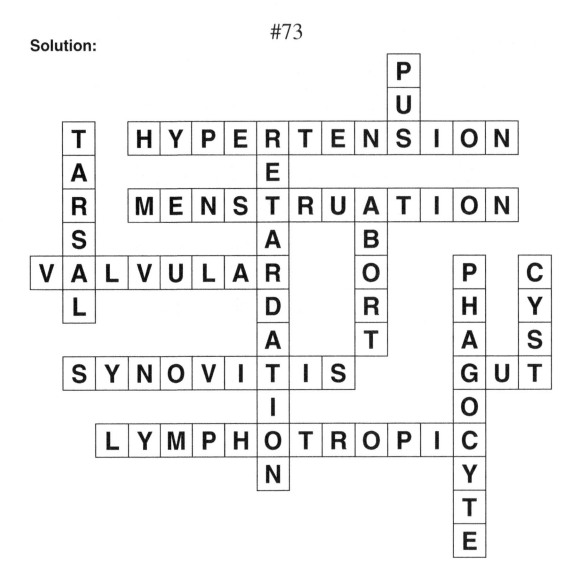

Solution:

```
M O T I L E                 L       M Y O M   Q
                                                U A D
O         F I B R O M Y O M A                   U
R         F           R                 D       A D                 M
I         L           D       S         R       U                   Y
B   E R U C T         O       E         U       P                   E
U         R           S       P         L       E                   N
N         A   Q U I N T U P L E T               R                   T
D         G           S       U                 E                   E
          G           S       T                 T                   R
      T E N T                 P                                     I
                              L                                     C
                  R O N G E U R
                              T
```

MOTILE
MORIBUND
FIBROMYOMA
QUADRUPLET
LORDOSIS
MYENTERIC
ERUCT
EFFLURAGE
SEPTUPLET
QUINTUPLET
TENT
RONGEUR

Solution:

```
                I N T E R C O S T A L
                        C
            P           H
            Y       U R O L A G N I A
            O           E
            R           G
            R           L
        T H A N A T O L O G Y
            E           B
            A   T E L E K I N E S I S
                        N
```

Made in the USA
Las Vegas, NV
27 September 2021

31203236R00083